Hair
Problems
Everyone has them

◆ *Dr Lim Kah-Beng*

TIMES BOOKS INTERNATIONAL
Singapore • Kuala Lumpur

© 1991 Times Editions Pte Ltd
Published by Times Books International
an imprint of Times Editions Pte Ltd
Times Centre
1 New Industrial Road
Singapore 1953

All illustrations by the author
All photographs courtesy of Shering-Plough Sdn. Bhd.

Times Subang
Lot 46, Subang Hi-Tech Industrial Park
Batu Tiga
40000 Shah Alam
Selangor Darul Ehsan
Malaysia

Reprinted 1995

Printed in Singapore

ISBN 981-204-440-X

CONTENTS

PREFACE

Hair loss is a distressing condition and many sufferers seek so-called "cures" which are not only expensive but often ineffective as well. There are so many "pseudo experts" and countless "hair-growth restorers" that medical education is necessary to help the desperate sufferer make the right decisions about treatment.

Unfortunately, doctors seldom have time to go into the intricacies of hair loss and its treatment. This is where this book may be helpful. It will help you understand hair loss, its causes and the treatments available. It will debunk many of the existing myths and eliminate the anxieties they often cause. In the long run, it will help you save a lot of money.

As a dermatologist, I see many types of patients with "hair loss." Some have genuine hair loss, but others turn out to be no more than over-anxious individuals with hairs and scalps that are quite normal.

But before going further, let me define what is meant by

hair loss. It means the shedding of hair together with its root. Hair that is lost without its root indicates breakage, not true hair loss.

The medical term for hair loss is alopecia. It is derived from "alopex," a Greek word meaning fox. Presumably, this is because the fox sheds its hair.

This book will provide you with some simple tests to detect early hair loss. Additionally, it will discuss ways of coping with some of the psychological problems that hair loss causes. All this will be done in a simple, non-technical language so that you won't go bald reading it!

1

COPING WITH HAIR LOSS

Hair loss has different effects on people. Some become extremely depressed, even suicidal; others are not the least bit concerned. What is important is not the hair loss itself but our reaction to it.

Obviously a person who regards his appearance to be the focus of his life will feel more stress than someone who doesn't consider it to be so. Some people have even used baldness to their advantage. Telly Savalas, of Kojak fame, and Yul Brynner are names that spring to mind. However, many find hair loss rather difficult to handle.

Fortunately for these, there is now treatment for some types of baldness. Even male pattern baldness (*androgenetic alopecia*), which was previously considered untreatable, now has treatment in the form of minoxidil lotion (see chapter 5). Although minoxidil does not cure all cases of male pattern baldness, it does help some patients regrow hair and may prevent further hair loss if used regularly.

Additionally, some types of baldness, no matter how bad

they look, are only temporary. *Telogen effluvium* (see chapter 7), for example, only causes temporary hair loss, and regrowth is the rule. And while hair is slowly growing back, there are now very well-made and attractive wigs to camouflage baldness and increase the person's self confidence. Let me relate some of my experiences to illustrate how hair loss affects some people and how stress may cause hair loss.

Thirty-year-old Kate came to my clinic angry and agitated. Quite understandably, I thought, because she was suffering from severe *alopecia areata* (a type of patchy hair loss) and was not responding to medical treatment. However, I also found that it wasn't because she was not getting better but that no one, including her doctors, cared to listen to what she was trying to say.

Kate thought her husband no longer found her attractive. As a result, she became depressed and kept to herself most of the time. What she needed was not more medication but a frank discussion with her husband.

I persuaded her to bring her husband the next time. She did and it became clear that her husband had actually been very understanding and supportive, and even encouraged her to purchase a wig so that she could go out like she used to. He still loved her, but had not reassured her of his affection, something she needed badly.

Kate had projected her own misplaced feelings onto her husband. The discussion benefitted her immensely. Thereafter, she felt happier and started wearing her wig and socializing again. I prescribed a steroid cream and saw her at regular intervals. Kate was a changed person. She was extremely talkative and what was most interesting was that her hair was growing back. I'm quite sure it wasn't the cream but the allaying of her fears that did the trick.

Michael, 35, came to my clinic regarding some rashes on the body. Examination showed that he had a fungal infection. He also had severe male pattern baldness which produced a very conspicuous patch of baldness on the crown and very deeply-receding temples.

I asked if he was concerned about the baldness to which he replied, "I'm not really ... I've had this for several years and it doesn't bother me." I just gave Michael some cream for the fungal infection.

Nine-year-old Maria was brought to my clinic by her mother because of a bald patch on the scalp. Examination showed a patch of broken hairs with stubbled ends, suggesting that she had been pulling her hair out.

After gentle questioning, she admitted to this. She couldn't help it. Maria had *trichotillomania* (*Tricho* means hair in Greek; *tillo* means to pull out; *mania* means compulsion), a compulsive hair-pulling disorder.

It became apparent that she began her hair-pulling habit after her family moved out of her grandmother's house. She was very attached to her grandmother and was very upset when she had to move away. An agreement was reached between Maria and her parents; she should spend one weekend a month at her grandmother's house. Her hair-pulling habit stopped after that.

Jennifer, 25, started losing large clumps of hair about two months after her father passed away. Examination revealed that she suffered from telogen effluvium. I reassured her that her hair loss was caused by bereavement and that her hair would grow back after six months or so. In the meantime, I advised her to wear a wig. I saw her at regular intervals after that and there were signs of regrowth after about three months. After six months, most of her hair had regrown and she was able to do without the wig.

Some, like Michael, are able to accept hair loss; others like Kate may suffer a variety of psychological reactions as well as from stress. This has to be dealt with because it may lead to more severe problems as well as related illnesses like stomach ulcers, irritable bowel and heart disease.

Stress may itself cause hair loss, as in the cases of Maria, who developed trichotillomania, and Jennifer, who developed telogen effluvium after her father's death. Telogen effluvium is usually temporary and hair regrows when the precipitating stress passes off. If the original stressful factor is replaced by another form of stress, then regrowth may be prevented or delayed.

Hair loss, admittedly, is very stressful but it is important not to let stress reach extreme proportions. If permitted, it can lead to a vicious hair-loss cycle or a stress-related illness. It is important to avoid this by learning how to manage stress better. Below are some methods of stress reduction you might like to consider.

Relaxation procedures

Autogenic Relaxation (self-induced relaxation). Lie comfortably in a quiet room. Close your eyes and breathe in and out. Focus on the breathing and try to relax at the same time. Say to yourself, "my head is getting heavier and warmer" and feel your head getting heavy and warm.

Move on to the left shoulder, then the left arm and the fingers. Do the same with the other side and then the legs. The sequence is not important. When you have finished, breathe in and out for a few minutes and then open your eyes. Repeat the procedure until you feel relaxed.

Tension-relaxation Exercise. Take a deep breath, tense the muscles of your body for a few seconds and then suddenly relax, breathing out at the same time. Do this several times.

Deep Breathing. Breathe deeply from the abdomen. This increases oxygen to the brain and relaxes the nerves.

Imagery. View pictures in your mind that will relax you. Try other forms of exercise too, like *taiji* and meditation.

Exercise

Exercise causes the body to release stress-reducing chemicals and this helps to calm the nerves. It doesn't matter what type of exercise it is, as long as you enjoy doing it and can keep up the momentum. But don't get competitive because this causes stress.

Make time for fun

Schedule time for recreation and take vacations. These help you to relax by temporarily diverting the mind away from the problem.

Make time for rest and sleep

All of us push ourselves a little too hard sometimes; our bodies and minds, in particular, need some rest. Vacations, short rests and even cat-naps help to reduce stress.

Talk to others

It helps to talk your problems through with others. You can talk to a close friend, relative, counsellor or even your family doctor. In some countries, people have gotten together to form organizations which provide education and psychological support for their members. You might like to start one.

Check off your tasks

Are you trying to do too many things at the same time? Make a list of the things you have to do and do them one at a time, ticking each off as it is completed.

If these measures do not help, approach your doctor. Your problems won't go away by just hoping or pretending they are not serious. They only get worse and make it even more difficult to manage. The following are some danger signs that indicate the need to get professional help:

- Persistent sadness or a feeling of hopelessness
- Irritability
- Anxiety and panic attacks
- Insomnia
- Inability to concentrate
- Low energy
- Inability to enjoy social or sexual activities
- Increased consumption of alcohol
- Use of drugs
- Suicidal thoughts

It must not be forgotten that education is a very important component of stress management. Misinformation and fear cause stress. Learning the truth about hair loss will help eliminate this. Education also helps you to discern between potentially useful remedies and those which are useless and a waste of money. So, read on.

2

QUESTIONS AND ANSWERS

There are many myths and misconceptions about hair loss. Apart from causing unnecessary anxiety, these are harmful because they may prevent you from seeking proper treatment or cause you to seek ineffective, expensive and, sometimes, harmful ones. Let us examine some questions commonly asked by patients, and, in the process, correct some misconceptions about hair loss and its treatment.

Is hair loss caused by taking a poor diet?
Poor nutrition will certainly starve the hair follicles of essential nutrients and cause hair loss. However, this is unusual in developed countries and those with high standards of living.

In these countries, it is not that we do not take enough food but rather that we do not take a well-balanced meal. We rely too much on fast foods and snacks. Thus, while we may be taking a lot of food, these may be lacking in vitamins and essential nutrients.

Admittedly, few people ever lose hair as a result of poor eating habits, but this does not mean that such habits should be encouraged. On the contrary, if you have hair loss, you should make a determined attempt to ensure that you take sufficient nutrients. You can achieve this by taking a well-balanced diet comprising of food from the four main food groups:

- Milk and dairy products
- Meat, poultry and fish
- Cereals and grains
- Vegetables and fruits

Many people make the mistake of taking specific vitamins, minerals or amino acids (see below). This is unnecessary and may lead to side effects. It is more important that you take a well-balanced diet.

Self-imposed starvation or crash diets rather than inadequate nutrition is another cause of hair loss in societies with high standards of living.

Do vitamin supplements help hair growth?
The food we take are complex molecules which have to be broken down into simpler ones before our body can utilize them. This is done by enzymes, and an important component of these enzymes are substances known as vitamins.

Vitamins are essential to life and health. It is not surprising, therefore, that they have been peddled as cures for anything from the simple cold to hair loss. Vitamin B-complex (so called because there are several B vitamins) in particular has been recommended for treating hair loss. Biotin and inositol belong to the B-complex group.

Biotin deficiency has been reported to cause hair loss in animals and there has been a case of a mentally-retarded boy developing baldness after taking two raw eggs a day for five years (raw egg white contains avidin, which binds strongly to biotin and prevents its absorption). This has led people to recommend taking biotin for hair loss. However, biotin is present in food items such as Brewer's yeast, liver, kidney and egg yolk and is also produced by intestinal bacteria so that deficiency is most unlikely to occur.

Inositol deficiency has also been reported to cause hair loss in animals and has, likewise, been recommended for hair loss. However, inositol deficiency is also unusual because it, too, is found in the food that we take. Citrus fruits (with the exception of lemon), cantaloupes, beans, grains and nuts are rich in inositol.

The amount of biotin and inositol required is actually very small; taking these specially and in large quantities is unnecessary and may even be harmful.

Vitamin A, for example, is also important for the hair's health. However, excessive intake of vitamin A can actually cause hair loss. The key is moderation, and a well balanced diet ensures the right amount of vitamins without the risk of overdosage.

Do minerals such as zinc help hair loss?
Iron deficiency can cause a diffuse hair loss which can be corrected by taking iron supplements.

Deficiency of other minerals are unusual under normal circumstances. Zinc deficiency may cause hair loss in babies who inherit an inability to absorb zinc, and adults who are on intravenous feeding (feeding through the veins). Normal individuals, however, receive more than enough zinc in the food that they take. Seafood and animal meats, whole grain products, wheat bran and germ and Brewer's yeast are all rich sources of zinc.

Zinc supplements have been given to patients with alopecia areata (patchy baldness), but the benefits are unconvincing. Moreover, the doses required for treatment often cause side effects such as nausea and may interfere with the absorption of other essential minerals such as copper. Generally, mineral supplements are unnecessary. Just take a well-balanced diet and rest assured that you will receive all the minerals necessary for hair growth.

Will taking amino acids induce hair growth?
Proteins are important for the growth of living cells, including those of the hair follicle. It is, therefore, important that we take sufficient amounts of proteins in our diets to help hair growth.

A well-balanced diet assures you of this. There is no advantage in taking specific amino acids which are merely simpler molecules of protein. Our body makes some of them and acquire others from the proteins that we eat.

Cysteine, a sulphur containing amino acid, is important for the sulphur bonds that give hair its strength and elasticity. It may be found in some over-the-counter medicines, but there is no proof at all that it helps hair growth.

Taking cysteine or any other amino acid is unnecessary because sufficient amounts of these are found in the proteins that we eat. Proteins from fish, meats, eggs and milk are rich in cysteine.

Does excessive sebum (oil) cause hair loss?
Oiliness of the scalp is due to the secretion of an oily

substance called sebum by the sebaceous (oil) glands in the scalp. Sebum production is increased by androgens (male hormones) which both men and women produce. Male pattern baldness is also due to androgens. It is, therefore, not uncommon for people with male pattern baldness to also have oily scalps.

This may have led to the erroneous belief that oiliness causes hair to drop. There is absolutely no truth in the suggestion that hair loss is caused by excessive oil clogging up the hair follicles and suffocating them. The hair follicles do not breathe in the same way as the lungs. They receive all the oxygen they need from the blood vessels in the scalp.

Is hair loss a sign of venereal disease (VD)?
Secondary syphilis, a venereal disease, may cause a patchy ("moth-eaten") alopecia. It was relatively common in the past but this is no longer the case. Most patients with hair loss nowadays do not suffer from it or any other form of venereal disease.

Does dandruff cause hair loss?
Dandruff (see chapter 7) causes flaking and itchiness of the scalp. It is a very common condition and, not surprisingly, people with hair loss may also suffer from it. However, dandruff does not normally cause hair loss.

Are bald people more intelligent?
There is a belief that deep thinkers go bald because of the heavy traffic of ideas going through their brains. There is no truth in this. You might even know of a few balding individuals with below-average IQs.

Are bald people are more virile?
This, again, has no scientific basis.

Does frequent shampooing cause hair loss?
Using the wrong shampoo can certainly make hair dry, brittle, lustreless or limp, but it will not cause hair loss. The growing part of the hair—the follicle—lies embedded deep in the scalp, beyond the reach of shampoos. Shampooing does no harm even to people who are losing hair. Indeed, the right sort of shampoo (see chapter 10) keeps the hair clean, and clean hair looks thicker and healthier. It may even retard male pattern baldness by washing away androgens present in sebum (see page 58).

How effective are the hair-growth restorers and tonics found on department store and pharmacy shelves?
There are a few hundred, perhaps even thousands, such products which claim to help hair grow. As long as there are bald people who believe these claims, you will see these "secret" formulae in shops.

Some of these "work," but only because the hair loss was a self-limiting form, or because of what doctors call the "placebo effect." The placebo effect is very well-known in medicine. For example, coloured tablets are more "effective" than white ones and some colours are "better" than others.

The more impressive and elaborate the treatment program, the surroundings, the packaging, the advertisement or the more convincing the sales person, the greater the placebo effect.

The placebo effect can be very powerful, but after a while the person will begin to realize that there is no definite sign of improvement—he just feels better but does not look better. Unfortunately, he may have already spent a large sum of money.

The United States Food and Drug Administration or the FDA (the drug regulatory body which also oversees the sale of over-the-counter medicines) has been watching the sale of hair-growth restorers since the 1970s.

After nearly 20 years, the FDA recently came out with a ruling controlling the sale of these products. It was reported in the newspapers that manufacturers have to provide the FDA with proof of the products' safety and effectiveness before it can be sold as a hair-growth restorer in the country. Whether the FDA's action will be followed by other countries remains to be seen.

At the moment, the only product approved by the FDA for the treatment of hair loss is minoxidil lotion. This product has been shown in large-scale medical trials to improve male pattern baldness.

Minoxidil is actually a drug used for treating hypertension, but its side effect of increasing hair growth has been exploited for the treatment of male pattern baldness. Being a medical product, minoxidil can only be obtained with a doctor's prescription. More about minoxidil in chapter 5.

Does brushing or pulling the hair, standing on the head and sleeping head down on a slant board stimulate hair growth?
The underlying rationale of all these methods is to increase blood circulation to the scalp. However, it is the blood flow to the tiny blood vessels in the follicles that is vital to the health of the hair. It is hard to imagine that brushing and pulling the hair can achieve this.

At the very most, they might increase the circulation to

the larger blood vessels in the scalp. However, there is already more than adequate blood in these vessels. You only need to get a cut to see how profusely it bleeds!

Common sense will tell you that pulling the hair may be detrimental. Forget about old wives' tale that 100 strokes a day with the hair brush is good for the hair. Brushing the hair helps to spread oil throughout the hair, making it more lustrous. It is fine for people with normal hair but not for those already suffering from hair loss.

Does brushing massage the scalp and stimulate blood circulation? This is most unlikely, in my view. Brushing would have to be so vigorous to achieve this that it will probably cause more hair loss or even draw blood from the scalp!

What about scalp and neck massage?
There is no definite proof that massage helps hair growth, but this does not mean that massage is not beneficial.

Massage is certainly relaxing and it does a person tremendous good to have someone fuss over their hair. My advice, in this case, is: "If it feels good, have it." But go to a trained masseuse because an incorrectly performed scalp massage may cause hair breakage.

Various tonics and secret ingredients may be rubbed into the scalp during a massage, but I am rather sceptical about their usefulness. I feel that, if anything, it is the massage that helps rather than these things.

Can a professional hairdresser help to disguise hair loss?
Most certainly a good hairdresser can cut and style thinning hair in such a way that it can enhance what is left, or conceal balding areas.

Does wine and brandy help to stimulate hair growth?
Alcohol causes blood vessels to dilate. One old remedy for
hair loss consists of rubbing wine or brandy into the scalp.
It does not help. Wine and brandy are meant to be drunk,
not wasted on bald scalps.

Is taking too much salt or soya sauce harmful to the hair?
It is often said that taking too much salt or soya sauce,
which contains large quantities of salt, causes hair loss.
This is not true. However, too much salt in the diet does
cause hypertension (high blood pressure) in some people
and should be avoided.

Does monosodium glutamate (MSG) cause hair loss?
MSG is a flavouring agent commonly used in Chinese
cooking. It causes the Chinese Restaurant Syndrome, so
named because it was first reported in people who had
eaten in Chinese restaurants. This consists of headaches,
dizziness, burning sensation in the extremities and chest
pain, but not hair loss.

Does wearing hats cause hair loss?
Bald people often wear caps and hats to conceal baldness.
This may have led people to believe that they cause hair
loss. This is incorrect. Tight hats and caps may sometimes
cause hair breakage from friction but not true hair loss.

Is swimming pool water bad for hair?
Chlorine, used for treating water in the swimming pool,
softens the cuticle (the outer layer of hair), making hair
drier and more brittle. Hair breakage may occur but not
true hair loss. This can be avoided by wearing a water-tight

cap during swimming or washing off the chlorine thoroughly and using a conditioner afterwards.

Does shaving the scalp stimulate hair growth?
This again has no basis at all. In a 1970 issue of the *Journal of Investigative Dermatology*, an article entitled *Shaving and Hair Growth* reported that two doctors, Y.L. Lynfield and P. MacWilliams, have actually studied the effects of shaving by getting volunteers to shave only one leg regularly, and have observed no difference in the weight of hair produced, the thickness (diameter) of hair or the rate of growth between the shaven and unshaven sides.

Does masturbation and excessive sex cause hair loss?
Such beliefs were probably started to discourage young people from engaging in masturbation and promiscuity. There is no basis at all that they cause hair loss.

What should I do if I suspect that I am losing excessive amounts of hair?
Some types of hair loss are temporary and require no treatment while others need to be treated early to prevent permanent hair loss.

Only a doctor can diagnose your problem with certainty. If there is no treatment, he will tell you. It is better to learn the sad truth early than learn it after you have spent nearly all your savings unnecessarily. You can see your family doctor or a dermatologist (skin specialist). Hair is a part of the skin and dermatologists are the people who can give you excellent advice in this area.

3

THE TRUTH ABOUT HAIR

Hair is found in all areas of the skin with the exception of a few areas such as the palm of the hand, the soles of the feet and lips. It has biological as well as psychological functions, though the former is seldom appreciated.

The large sums of money people spend on hair care products and hairstyles, and the great anxiety they experience when they lose their hair, are an indication of the immense psychological value of hair.

Hair care is big business and so is hair loss. There is a wide range of hair products claiming to "nourish" or "feed" hair. And when hair falls out, there is an equally large number of products claiming to make hair grow again. Most of these claims have no basis at all. Read on to find out why.

This chapter will help you understand more about your hair and provide you with the basic information necessary to help you make the correct decision about treatment.

Types of hair

There are essentially three types of hair: *lanugo*, *vellus* and *terminal* hair.

Lanugo hair is the very fine, long, wispy, non-pigmented hair found on the unborn. It is shed inside the womb at about the seventh or eighth month of pregnancy, or soon after birth. Vellus hair covers the body surface after birth and is fine, soft, velvety and non-pigmented. The third type of hair is terminal hair, which is long, coarse and pigmented.

After puberty, vellus hair gives way to terminal hair on the face and chest in men, and the pubic area and armpits in both sexes. This change is brought about by androgens (male hormones) which both men and women have. Curiously, the same hormones can later cause terminal hair to revert back to vellus hair on the scalps of people with male pattern baldness (see chapter 5).

Hair structure and growth

The hair that you see on the skin is actually dead. The living portion of hair is the follicle which lies embedded in the dermis (Fig. 1). Let us examine the hair and its follicle to understand what hair is made of and how it grows.

Hair is comprised of three layers—an inner core called the *medulla*, an outer layer called the *cuticle* and a layer in between called the *cortex* (Fig. 2).

The medulla is composed of round cells and was at one time wrongly believed to be the lifeline of hair through which nutrients from the body reached all parts of the hair. This misconception even led to the practice of singeing the ends of hair to prevent the escape of "sap" from the medulla.

The outer layer, the cuticle, is composed of transparent

23

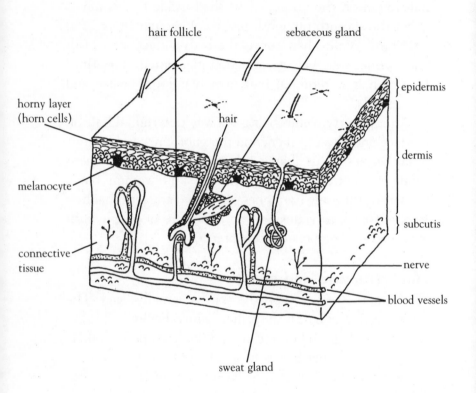

Fig. 1 Structure of normal skin

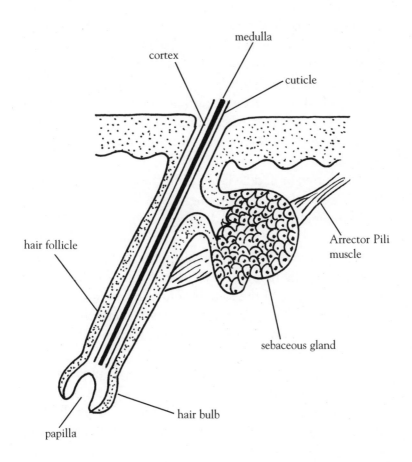

Fig. 2 Structure of Hair

overlapping cells and serves as a protective layer for hair. If the "imbrications" or the spaces between the overlapping layers of the cuticle are open, then hairs tend to get entangled. Alkaline substances such as soap tend to open the imbrications whereas acidic substances close them down (see chapter 10). Closed imbrications make hairs smooth and more manageable.

Indeed, the key to making hair look good is ensuring that the cuticle is in good condition. Most hair care products affect the state of the cuticle and this is what hair care is really about.

The cortex or middle layer forms the greater part of hair. It is composed of tightly cemented cells and most of the hair's pigment, melanin. It also provides strength and elasticity to the hair.

Hair protrudes through small pores in the skin and is produced by the hair follicles embedded in the dermis (see Fig. 1). The base of the follicle comprises an inner portion known as the *hair bulb*, which contains actively-dividing cells. This surrounds another structure known as the *papilla* (see Fig. 2).

The papilla contains a rich network of blood vessels which supplies the actively-dividing cells of the hair bulb with essential nutrients. New cells produced by the hair bulb are pushed towards the surface by still newer cells coming from below.

As these cells move towards the surface, they accumulate into a hard substance called keratin and die. These dead keratin-laden cells form hair. Hair is, therefore, dead. It won't bleed, leak body fluids or hurt when cut. Keratin is also the same hard substance found in nails.

Halfway up the follicle is the arrector pili muscle.

Contraction of this muscle causes the hair to stand on end and form goose pimples. A sebaceous (oil) gland opens into the follicle just above the arrector pili muscle and produces an oily secretion called sebum. Sebum smoothens the overlapping cuticle cells, making hair shiny, smooth and less likely to get entangled. Too much sebum makes the scalp greasy.

The follicle goes through two main stages: *anagen* and *telogen*. There is also an intermediate stage called *catagen*, which lasts only a few weeks.

Anagen is the growth stage. During anagen, the hair bulb produces new cells and causes the hair to increase in length at a rate of half an inch per month.

The anagen stage lasts about five years (or a range of two to five years). Using these figures, we can calculate the maximum length hair will attain if it is not cut. Since hair grows half an inch a month for five years, the total length achieved will be 30 inches. However, some people have longer and some shorter anagen stages. People with longer anagen stages are able to grow longer hairs than others.

The length of anagen also varies according to the area of the skin. Eyebrow hair, for example, has a short anagen stage of three months. This is why eyebrow hair does not grow very long.

The other stage is the resting stage or telogen. This lasts about five months (or a range of two to five months). Hair stops growing and is shed at the end of it.

An average adult between the ages of 20 to 30 years has 100,000 hairs. Of these, about 15% are in telogen and the remaining 85% are in anagen. In other words, 15,000 hairs are in telogen. If we assume that telogen is five months or 150 days long, then we can expect to lose 100 hairs per day

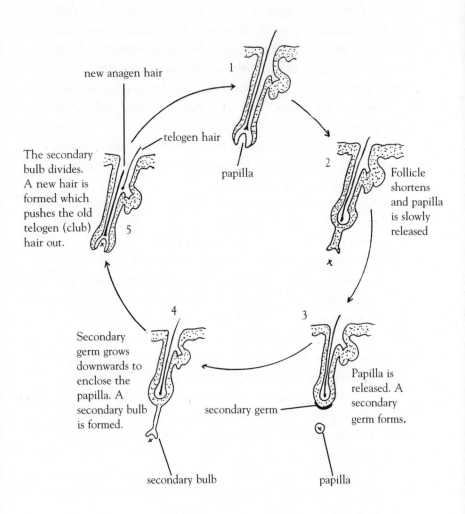

new anagen hair

1

telogen hair

The secondary
bulb divides.
A new hair is
formed which
pushes the old
telogen (club)
hair out.

5

papilla

2

Follicle
shortens
and papilla
is slowly
released

4

Secondary
germ grows
downwards to
enclose the
papilla. A
secondary bulb
is formed.

secondary germ

secondary bulb

3

Papilla is
released. A
secondary
germ forms.

papilla

Fig. 3 Hair cycle

(15,000 hairs divided by 150 days). This is why it is often said that a normal person can lose up to 100 hairs per day. However, this figure is merely a guide because the proportion of hairs in telogen and the duration of telogen varies from person to person. The normal range of hair loss varies from 50 to 100 per day.

In humans, the follicles develop out of phase with one another; meaning some hairs are falling while others are growing. This ensures that there is always hair on the scalp.

In some animals, the follicle develops in phase with each other in certain regions of the skin. At the end of telogen, the entire area becomes devoid of hair. This results in seasonal shedding of the hair. A similar situation may occur in humans when the follicles are prematurely pushed into telogen. Such a situation may occur after extreme stress, childbirth or surgery. This condition is known as telogen effluvium (see chapter 7).

The sheep is an interesting animal. Its hair follicles are always in anagen and hair keeps on growing longer and longer, until cut. Unfortunately, our scalp hairs do not behave in the same way. Otherwise, we would not have to contend with some forms of baldness.

Fig. 3 shows the follicle in different stages of development. The follicle is longest during anagen and shortens gradually until it reaches telogen. As the follicle shortens, the papilla becomes separated from the hair bulb. Below the hair bulb, a secondary germ forms. This divides to form a new bulb which grows downwards and encloses the papilla, forming a new follicle. The new follicle enters anagen and the cells of the hair bulb divide to form a new hair. The growth of the new hair dislodges the old telogen hair.

You should now understand the structure of hair and its

growth cycle. Because the protruding hair is dead, no amount of nourishment poured onto it will make any difference. The growing portion of hair is the follicle which receives its nourishment from the blood vessels in the papilla— meaning, from the inside rather than from the outside. This is why rubbing nutrients on the scalp does not make sense. However, the dead cells of the hair allows it to be cut, remodelled and coloured to whatever colour you desire without causing any pain or discomfort.

Variations in hair

The colour of hair, its shape and quantity varies from individual to individual. Some have black hair, some red, some blonde, curly, straight, thick and thin. All these characteristics are determined by genetic or racial factors.

Straight hair is round in cross-section and arises more or less perpendicular to the skin surface. Curly hair is oval and grows out at an angle, twisting and curling as it grows. Each type has its advantages and disadvantages.

Straight hair is easy to manage, but rather ordinary looking. This is why people like to wave their hair. Curly hair is attractive but not when the curls are too tight. Tightly curled hair is very difficult to manage and this is one reason why some people have their hair straightened.

Curly hair may sometimes turn back on itself and grow back into the skin, or it may puncture the follicle instead of growing out. The hair is said to be in-grown. In-grown hairs irritate the skin, causing it to become inflamed. They usually occur over the back of the neck where pressure from collars encourage hairs to turn back into the skin.

Another very rare type of hair is known as woolly hair— it feels and looks like wool. Woolly hair is flat or kidney-shape in cross-section.

Hair colour is determined in a complex manner by the genes we inherit from our parents. It has mostly to do with the melanin (a skin pigment) in hair. There are two types of melanin: eumelanin, which is black and gives black or brown hair; and phaemelanin, which is red or yellow and gives auburn or blonde hair. However, the ultimate colour of hair depends not only on the type of melanin, but also the shape and position of the melanin granules within the hair and the way air bubbles within the cortex refract light.

Asians and blacks have black hair while Caucasians have a wide variety of hair colours. The colour, thickness and quantity of hair are inter-related. Light-coloured hair such as blonde hair is finer and denser whereas red and black hair is thicker but less dense.

The number of hair follicles and hair decreases as a person ages. An adult scalp 20-30 years old has about 615 follicles per square centimetre of scalp. This falls to about 485 when the person is 30-50 years old, and 435 when the person is 80-90 years old.

As the number of follicles decrease, so will the number of hairs. Therefore, it is normal for hair to thin as we grow older and there is no treatment that will permanently reverse this process.

4

WHAT MAY AFFECT HAIR LOSS

In chapter 3, you learnt some facts about the structure of hair, its growth and its variations in colour, shape and density. You also discovered that genes have a lot to do with these characteristics. But there are other factors as well which may affect your hair. Let us take a closer look at all these factors.

Genes

Genes determine the shape of our hair, its colour, thickness and density and how fast or long it grows. The genes that control these characteristics are inherited from each parent.

Genes, you will learn in the next chapter, also determine whether you are going to be susceptible to male pattern baldness (androgenetic alopecia) or not.

There are also some congenital types of baldness (that is, baldness present from birth) and structural abnormalities of the hair which are inherited.

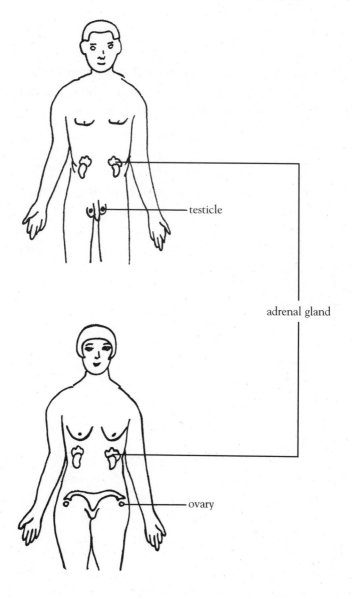

testicle

adrenal gland

ovary

Fig. 4 Sites of androgen production

Race

Some races are more prone than others to develop male pattern baldness. Caucasians are particularly prone and may develop very severe forms of male pattern baldness; Blacks are less prone and Orientals the least prone.

Sex

Hair grows faster in women than men—a good excuse for women if their menfolk complain of their frequent visits to the hairdresser! Women also have more problems with hair breakage because of damage from bleaching, permanent waving and styling. However, women are protected by female hormones and tend to have less severe male pattern baldness (see chapter 5).

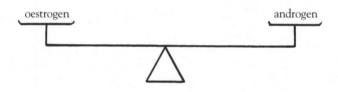

Fig. 5 Oestrogen and androgen have opposing actions on the hair follicle

Hormones

Androgens, the male hormones present in both men and women, are believed to be the main cause of male pattern baldness in a genetically predisposed person. Fig. 4 shows the sites of androgen production in men and women.

Oestrogen, female hormones produced by the ovaries, counteracts the effects of androgens (Fig. 5). This is why women tend to have less severe male pattern baldness than men. The only exception is in women who produce excess androgens. These women not only have severe male pattern baldness, but also hirsutism (excessive and coarse facial hair), severe acne, menstrual disturbances and infertility.

Androgens are necessary in order for male pattern baldness to develop. If androgen production is cut off by castration, males will not develop male pattern baldness at all. However, given the choice of a good sex life or baldness, I have no doubt which men would chose!

Other hormones may also affect hair. Lack of the pituitary hormones or too much or too little thyroid hormones can cause diffuse thinning of the hair. A transient deficiency of thyroid hormones may also contribute to the hair loss that occurs after pregnancy (see next section).

Pregnancy and childbirth

The increase in nutrition and hormones necessary to support pregnancy also affects the hair. During pregnancy, anagen (growing stage) is maintained for longer than normal and about 95% of the hairs are in anagen. After delivery, nutrition and hormone levels return to normal and the hair becomes somewhat starved. This causes the hair to go into telogen (resting stage).

Since more hair was in anagen to begin with, more will also move into telogen. These telogen hairs are shed at the end of telogen, two to five months later. This condition is known as telogen effluvium. Telogen effluvium after pregnancy is self-limiting and hair grows to its normal state after six months or so.

Another cause of hair loss after pregnancy is hypothyroidism (lack of thyroid hormones). This is known to cause diffuse thinning of the hair. About 10% of pregnant women develop a transient thyroid deficient state after delivery and this may account for some of the hair loss. However, thyroid levels return to normal after six months and so does the hair.

Iron requirements increase during pregnancy and iron deficiency may develop if dietary intake is insufficient. This may also cause a diffuse thinning of the hair. However, iron deficiency during pregnancy is uncommon because most women take iron supplements during pregnancy or take enough iron in their diet.

Birth control pills

The most popular birth control pills are the combined pills which contain an oestrogen and a progestogen (a synthetic progesterone). Oestrogen and progesterone are female hormones.

Birth control pills prevents pregnancy by making the body believe it is pregnant. The effect of this on hair is more or less the same as in a true pregnancy, that is, anagen is prolonged. When you stop taking the pills, large quantities of anagen hairs are pushed into telogen and this is followed by a telogen effluvium two to five months later.

A second form of hair loss can also occur. The combined pill can be classified into oestrogen-dominant and androgen-dominant pills. Androgen-dominant pills contain progestogens which have androgenic properties. Women taking these pills may sometimes develop male pattern baldness if they happen to be genetically predisposed. Check with the pharmacist or your doctor if you are not sure.

Menopause

The ovaries that produce female hormones become inactive after menopause and the protection of oestrogens is lost. Androgens are not affected because they are still produced by the adrenal glands which sit on top of the kidneys. The unopposed action of androgens cause many women to develop male pattern baldness after menopause.

Age

The number of hair follicles and hair falls with age from puberty onwards. When a person is 20-30 years old, there are about 615 follicles per square centimetre on his scalp. By the ages of 30-50 years, this falls to 485. By 80-90 years, it becomes 435 per square centimetre. Thinning of the hair, therefore, occurs as part of the ageing process.

Iron deficiency

Insufficient intake of iron in the diet may cause diffuse thinning of the hair. The iron in vegetables is inferior compared to that in meat and strict vegetarians may suffer from iron deficiency.

Iron deficiency may also develop during pregnancy if intake is insufficient (see pregnancy and childbirth). Chronic blood loss from any cause, like bleeding ulcers, haemorrhoids (piles) and heavy periods may also lead to iron deficiency. This can be detected through a blood test.

Diet

Protein malnutrition may cause alterations in hair colour and texture, and increased hair loss. However, this is uncommon in countries with high standards of living. The more likely cause of diet-related hair loss in these countries is not malnutrition but self-imposed crash diets.

Self-imposed starvation deprives the hairs of essential nutrients and cause them to go into telogen (resting stage). This is followed by telogen effluvium two to five months later.

Stress

Sudden, severe emotional stress can precipitate telogen effluvium or alopecia areata (see chapter 6), but it is not clear whether chronic stress can also aggravate an existing hair loss problem.

But why take chances? Reducing stress will certainly not make hair loss worse and may even help. Moreover, stress can cause other problems such as tension headaches, digestive problems, stomach ulcers and heart attacks. Reducing stress is undoubtedly a good thing. Simple methods of stress reduction were described in chapter 1.

Stress may affect hair in another way. Some people have a habit of twirling or biting their hair. This can cause hair loss or breakage.

Trichotillomania, a compulsive hair-pulling disorder that usually affects children and women, is also due to underlying emotional stress (Fig. 6). Maria, the girl mentioned earlier, suffered from this condition (p. 8).

On the other hand, there are some people who complain of "hair loss" but show no evidence of it, or at least no greater thinning than their contemporaries. These individuals may suffer from a disturbance of body image.

This condition, known medically as *dysmorphophobia*, was described by English dematologist Dr John A. Cotterill. He described it to be a symptom of underlying psychiatric diseases such as depression, which require treatment.

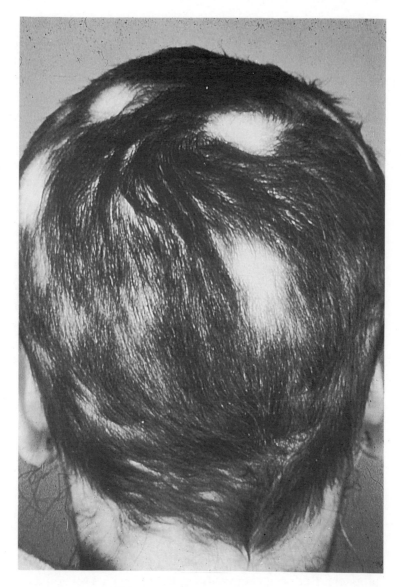

Fig. 6   Hair-pulling alopecia

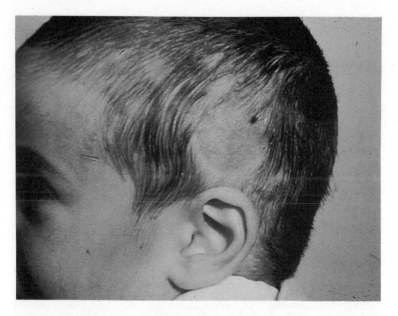

Fig. 7   Inflamed lesion in a young boy

Friction

Friction from tight hair bands, wigs and hats can sometimes cause hair to break. In infants, hair loss may occur as a rim along the back of the head due to friction from the pillow case or crib sheet before the baby is able to lift its head. The hairs are telogen hairs which are destined to be shed. The hair loss is, therefore, harmless and temporary.

Pressure

Prolonged pressure on one area of the scalp during long medical operations that exceed four hours may cause alopecia. Redness, oozing and crusting appears several days after the operation, and this is followed by hair loss the next month. It is due to reduced blood flow to the hair follicles in the region. This is temporary.

Massage

Improper and overvigorous scalp massage may cause hair to break, adding another problem to hair loss.

Hairstyles

Permanent waves, frequent bleaching, the use of hot combs and hair straighteners may damage the hair and cause breakage. Corn-rowing, tight braiding, buns, tight curlers and ponytails can also pull hair out by the roots and cause a type of alopecia known as traction alopecia. This characteristically affects the front and temples.

Infection

Ringworm of the scalp (*tinea capitis*) typically produces red scaly bald patches with broken-off hair stumps (Fig. 7). Children are more commonly affected.

A very severe form of tinea capitis may be caused by animal fungi. It results in a large, painful abscess called a kerion. Kerions may cause severe scarring and permanent hair loss. Fungal infections can be confirmed by microscopic examination and culture (growth) of specimens of hair. The treatment is with oral and applied anti-fungal medication.

Bacterial folliculitis (an infection of the hair follicles) may also cause hair loss. If severe, scarring and permanent baldness may result; early treatment with oral antibiotics helps prevent this.

Secondary syphilis may cause a patchy "moth-eaten" type of alopecia. The diagnosis can be confirmed with the Venereal Disease Reference Laboratory (or VDRL) blood test. Hair regrows after treatment.

Fever

Prolonged fever caused by infections such as malaria and typhoid can also cause telogen effluvium.

Drugs

A number of drugs have been reported to cause hair loss. These include blood-thinning drugs such as warfarin, heparin and phenindione; anti-thyroid drugs such as thiouracil and carbimazole; and anti-cancer drugs such as cyclophosphamide, adriamycin and vincristine.

Excessive intake of vitamin A also causes hair loss. Roaccutane (13 cis-retinoic acid), a vitamin-A derivative used for the treatment of severe acne, can also cause hair loss which is reversible when intake is stopped. Birth control pills are another cause of drug-induced hair loss.

Skin diseases

Skin diseases such as discoid lupus erythematosus, lichen planus and scleroderma may affect the scalp and cause scarring and permanent hair loss.

These conditions can be confirmed with a scalp biopsy (see page 82). Early treatment is necessary because scarring can completely destroy the hair follicles, eliminating all chances of regrowth.

Cancers

Underlying cancers, particularly Hodgkin's lymphoma (a cancer of the lymph glands), are another rare cause of diffuse hair loss.

5

MALE PATTERN BALDNESS

Male pattern baldness is a form of baldness which affects most men and some women. It is also known as common baldness or androgenetic alopecia, a name which suggests it has something to do with androgens and genes.

Male pattern baldness may be due to three factors:

Androgens

Androgens are influential for the following reasons.

Women who produce excess androgens can develop very severe male pattern baldness. It has also been found that the hair follicles of individuals with male pattern baldness convert circulating androgens to more potent androgens at a faster rate than normal follicles. These androgens accumulate in the skin and cause the hair follicles there to regress.

Male pattern baldness develops as a result of this. The increase in androgens occurs locally, which is why many individuals with male pattern baldness have normal levels of circulating androgens, and women with male pattern baldness still look feminine and can conceive and have babies normally.

The importance of androgens is further illustrated by the following report by Dr James B. Hamilton of the State University Medical Center in New York City in the *American Journal of Anatomy*. In an identical twin study, one twin who had been castrated before puberty retained all his hair at 40 but his uncastrated twin brother had slowly become bald. When the castrated twin was treated with testosterone (an androgen), he became as bald as his twin brother within six months.

Genes

Genes are the blueprints of our body, and several thousands of these can be found on paired structures called chromosomes.

We inherit one chromosome from each of our parents. Many of our characteristics such as the colour of our hair and eyes, height and facial appearance are inherited. This is why there is often a resemblance between family members.

The tendency to develop male pattern baldness is also believed to be inherited. According to one theory, men who inherit one or both genes for male pattern baldness will develop it whereas only women who inherit both genes are affected.

Genetic Make-up	Men	Women
Bb	Bald	Normal
BB	Bald	Bald
bb	Normal	Normal

(where B is the gene for male pattern baldness.)

However, not everyone agrees with this theory and it is likely that the genetics of male pattern baldness is much more complex.

The importance of inheritence is illustrated by Dr Hamilton's observations that a eunuch with normal male relatives did not develop male pattern baldness, whereas one whose male relatives were affected tended to develop male pattern baldness when treated with the same amount of androgens.

Age

Male pattern baldness becomes more common as a person ages. Significant male pattern baldness, defined as at least a deep receding of the front hairline, occurs in 5% of men under 20, 30% of men at the age of 30, and 50% of men at the age of 50.

You may recall that the number of hair follicles decreases with increasing age and hair becomes thinner as a result. It seems to affect the same areas affected by male pattern baldness, accentuating it.

Theoretically, male pattern baldness can occur at any age after puberty. In men, it commonly develops during the 20s and 30s. Women usually develop male pattern baldness after menopause unless they have inherited susceptible genes. If so, male pattern baldness may begin just as early.

Fortunately, male pattern baldness in women is never as severe as in men because the female hormone, oestrogen, counteracts the effect of androgens on the hair follicle. However, if it is severe in young women, this may indicate excess androgen secretion. Besides menstrual disturbances, these women usually suffer from infertility, hirsutism (excessive and coarse facial hair, particularly on the upper

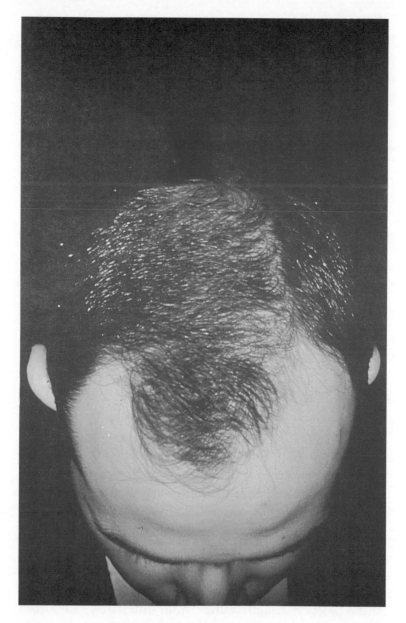

Fig. 8   Male pattern alopecia

lip, chin and cheeks), and severe acne. Hormone investigations need to be done.

In men, male pattern baldness usually begins as a receding hairline along the front and temples (Fig. 8) and then a thinning of the crown. In severe cases, these areas merge until only a horseshoe rim of hair remains on the sides and back.

Severe male pattern baldness in young men is, fortunately, not very common and affects only 2% of them by the time they reach 30. As explained earlier, severe male pattern baldness is not normally seen in women and the pattern of baldness is also different. Women usually develop diffuse thinning of the crown rather than a receding hair line. Figs. 9 and 10 illustrate the pattern of male pattern baldness in men and women.

In male pattern baldness, there is a reduction in the duration of anagen and a consequent increase in telogen hairs. This is reflected in a lower anagen:telogen (A:T) ratio. Shorter hairs are produced because of the shortened anagen stage. The hair follicle also shrinks in size over each successive hair cycle. Consequently, the hairs produced are finer and lighter in colour.

Initially, indeterminate hairs are produced. These are intermediate in length, thickness and colour between terminal and vellus hairs. Eventually, even these are reduced to a fluff. Another characteristic finding in male pattern baldness is the discovery of telogen hairs of different thickness. It is due to hair follicles of different sizes entering telogen.

You may recall that under the influence of androgens, vellus hair on some parts of the body such as the face, chest, armpits, and pubic region changes to coarse, pigmented

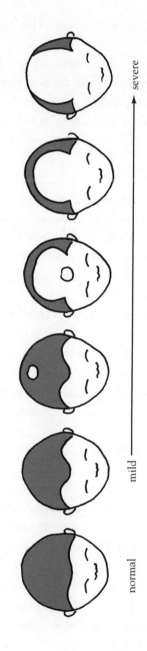

Fig. 9 Different severities of male pattern baldness in men

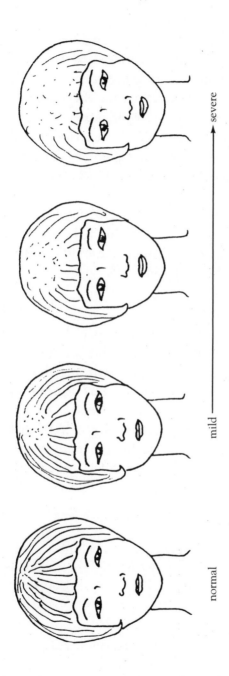

Fig. 10 Male pattern baldness in women

terminal hairs. On the scalps of individuals with male pattern baldness, however, the same androgens seem to do the opposite—cause terminal hairs to revert back to vellus hairs. That androgens should exert opposite effects on hairs on the scalp and hairs elsewhere is a paradox.

There is also racial variation in the severity of male pattern baldness. Caucasians, for example, have the most severe form of male pattern baldness. Blacks have less severe forms and Orientals the least.

Seborrhoea (increased sebum or oil production) often accompanies male pattern baldness. This is because the sebaceous glands are stimulated by the same androgens that cause male pattern baldness (see Fig. 11).

Diagnosis

The pattern of male pattern baldness is quite characteristic in men, but the diagnosis may be more difficult to make in women. A positive family history, if present, may help. If necessary, the diagnosis can be confirmed by determining the anagen:telogen (A:T) ratio.

The A:T ratio is normally at least 4:1, but in male pattern baldness, it is reduced in the areas that are affected by it. The presence of telogen hairs of different diameters also suggests male pattern baldness.

Treatment

Treatment is not necessary if male pattern baldness is mild and the person is not distressed by it. But the following treatments are available:

Minoxidil
Minoxidil is a drug used for the treatment of severe

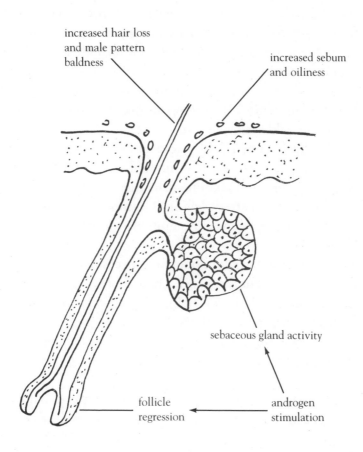

increased hair loss
and male pattern
baldness

increased sebum
and oiliness

sebaceous gland activity

follicle
regression

androgen
stimulation

Fig. 11 Androgen affects both the sebaceous gland
and hair follicle

hypertension (high blood pressure). One of its side effects is increased hair growth, often in unwanted places. However, its potential as a hair-growth restorer largely went unrecognized until Dr Anthony R. Zappacosta, an American cardiologist, reported in the *New England Journal of Medicine* that one of his patients, a bald man of 38, had experienced hair regrowth after treatment with minoxicil. Soon, dermatologists were dissolving minoxidil and applying the lotion on bald scalps.

Upjohn Company, the manufacturer of minoxidil, also started its own trials on minoxidil. Initial studies were conducted on stumped-tail macaque monkeys who also developed male pattern baldness during adolescence. The results were impressive; the animals started to grow new hair.

Subsequently, trials in human were conducted in several centres throughout the world. These more or less confirmed that 2% minoxidil lotion helps some cases of male pattern baldness affecting the crown.

However, the following points need to be emphasized about minoxidil:

1. Minoxidil lotion only helps male pattern baldness affecting the crown. It does not seem to help the receding hairline.
2. Not all patients respond to minoxidil lotion. The commonly quoted figure is 20-50% cosmetically acceptable improvement. The term "cosmetically acceptable" means a satisfactory improvement in appearance, not complete regrowth. In my experience, minoxidil does not produce complete regrowth. Some patients show dense regrowth, but this is rare and occurs

in less than 10% of cases.

3. Minoxidil works better in men below the age of 40 if the baldness is less than 10 years old, if the bald patch is less than 10 centimetres in diameter, or if there are more than 100 indeterminate hairs in a 2.5-centimetre diameter area in the centre of the bald area.

4. The minoxidil lotion has to be used for at least four months before signs of regrowth become visible. Perseverence is necessary during this period.

5. Maximum regrowth is seen at eight to 10 months, after which there is little improvement.

6. Once regrowth is achieved, minoxidil must be continued or the regrown hair will start to fall out. Minoxidil is expensive and the cost of treatment is considerable.

Minoxidil is no miracle drug, but it is the best treatment available for male pattern baldness. It is up to you to decide whether it is worth spending your money on it, keeping in view the above considerations.

Some studies have suggested that although minoxidil does not induce regrowth in some patients, it does appear to prevent further loss as long as it is used regularly. Minoxidil may therefore have a prophylactic (preventive) action against baldness. Again, the problem is cost.

However, minoxidil lotion appears to be safe to use on people with a normal heart. Systemic side effects such as lowered blood pressure and palpitations are uncommon because very little minoxidil is absorbed through the skin. Still, patients on it should have their blood pressure checked regularly.

Minoxidil should also not be used on scalps that are damaged by eczema or cuts because of the possibility of increased absorption through the damaged skin. Minor side effects such as itching, prickling and dryness of the skin and skin allergy may sometimes occur.

Minoxidil promotes hair growth by prolonging anagen (the growth stage). There are two possible mechanisms of action. Minoxidil reduces blood pressure by causing the blood vessels to dilate, and it has been suggested that the dilation of the small blood vessels in the papilla of the hair follicle stimulates hair growth.

Interestingly, another anti-hypertensive drug, diazozide, reduces blood pressure in the same way and also causes increased hair growth as a side effect. This theory presumes that male pattern baldness is partly due to a reduction of blood flow to the papilla, but this is unlikely because grafts of hair-bearing skin transplanted onto the bald areas do not start to lose hair, which it should do if the blood supply to the papilla is the determining factor.

The second mechanism is a direct stimulation of hair follicle cell growth. Experiments have confirmed that minoxidil can stimulate the division and prolong the survival of these cells. This, I feel, is the most likely mechanism.

Most of the published studies on minoxidil have involved men and the question on many people's minds has been: "Does minoxidil help male pattern baldness in women?"

Theoretically, at least, minoxidil should work but the question is how well. Unfortunately, this question cannot be answered at the moment because there is very little published data on the use of minoxidil in women with male pattern baldness.

There has also been a recent report that treatment with low concentration minoxidil and tretinoin is even more effective (see next page).

Topical tretinoin

Tretinoin is a vitamin-A derivative originally developed for the treatment of acne (pimples). It is known to stimulate the division of epithelial cells and also promotes the formation of new blood vessels in the skin.

Tretinoin has aroused great interest recently because it was reported to delay skin ageing and reverse early wrinkles. There has been a report by Dr Gail Bazzano and her colleagues in New Orleans which suggests that tretinoin lotion also stimulates hair growth. The investigators treated patients with 0.5% minoxidil, 0.025% tretinoin, a combination of both drugs, and placebo (dummy drug). No hair growth was observed with minoxidil (however, note that this is lower than the 2% concentration recommended for male pattern baldness) or placebo, but 58% of the patients treated with tretinoin showed signs of regrowth.

Regrowth was even more impressive with the combination of minoxidil and tretinoin—66% responded positively. This study suggests that tretinoin has potential as a hair-growth restorer and is particularly effective when combined with a low concentration of minoxidil. This is certainly interesting but needs further confirmation.

Cyclical anti-androgen therapy

Oestrogen, you may remember, protects against male pattern baldness whereas androgens encourage it. It has been combined with anti-androgens to block the effects of androgens on the hair follicle to treat male pattern baldness.

The anti-acne drug, Diane, combines ethinyl oestradiol (an oestrogen) with cyproterone acetate (an anti-androgen) and has been reported to induce hair growth in some women with male pattern baldness. It cannot be used in men because of the risk of feminization.

Some dermatologists feel that the dose of cyproterone acetate in Diane is too low and usually give patients an extra tablet of cyproterone acetate.

Steroid-oestrogen therapy

This involves the use of a steroid like prednisolone and an oestrogen. Prednisolone suppresses the production of androgens by the adrenal glands and oestrogen counteracts the effects of androgens on the hair follicle. This form of treatment has been reported to help some women. Unfortunately, it is also unsuitable for men because of the risk of feminization.

Topical (applied) oestrogen and progesterone

Oestrogen and progesterone are female sex hormones. Topical oestrogen works by inhibiting androgen production, but this may have undesirable effects in men.

Topical progesterone has been advocated on the basis that application to the pubic skin of normal males inhibited the conversion of testosterone to DHT (a potent androgen). It may retard the progression of male pattern baldness.

Topical anti-androgens

Anti-androgens block the effect of androgens on the hair follicle. However, they cause feminization when taken orally. Topical (applied) anti-androgens have been used instead in men, but the results have not been encouraging.

One topical anti-androgen, 11 alpha-hydroxypro-gesterone, has been reported to have an effect, but this was based on very fine measurements such as the diameter of the hair shaft rather than observable regrowth (which is important when dealing with a cosmetic problem). Nonetheless, this is a very promising area for research and it is possible that an effective topical anti-androgen will eventually be found.

Spironolactone

This is an oral drug used for treating water retention or oedema. It also has anti-androgenic properties and has been reported to help women with male pattern baldness.

However, spironolactone commonly causes menstrual irregularities in women if taken on its own. This can be avoided by taking a combined birth control pill during the first 21 days of a 28-day menstrual cycle. Spironolactone cannot be used in men because it causes gynaecomastia (breast enlargement).

Cimetidine

This is an oral, anti-ulcer drug which also has anti-androgenic properties. It has been reported to help a few women with male pattern baldness. However, cimetidine is also known to cause hair loss as a side effect. This seems strange for a drug that is supposed to help hair grow. Other side effects include diarrhoea, rashes and dizziness.

Cyclosporin

It suppresses the body's immune system and is used to prevent the rejection of transplanted organs. It promotes hair growth as a side effect and has been reported to induce regrowth in some patients with alopecia areata.

There has also been a report of a male patient regrowing hair while taking cyclosporin. It may work by directly stimulating hair follicle cell growth. Unfortunately, cyclosporin is rather toxic (especially to the kidneys) when taken orally, so doctors have tried to overcome this by applying it externally instead. Unfortunately, the results have been disappointing, probably because topical cyclosporin has difficulty penetrating the skin and cannot reach the follicles. Doctors are still trying out different formulations of topical cyclosporin to overcome this.

Diazozide
This is another drug used for treating hypertension. Like minoxidil, it too causes the blood vessels to dilate (thus lowering blood pressure) and hair growth as a side effect.

Trials are already in progress to determine the effectiveness of topical diazozide in the treatment of male pattern baldness. Its manufacturer, Schering USA, is rather tight lipped about the results and any information apart from the fact that trials were in progress could not be obtained. It remains to be seen whether topical diazozide will eventually prove to be effective.

Cosmetic therapy
This includes creative hair styles, wigs and surgery to disguise hair loss. More about them in chapters 9 and 10.

People suffering from hair loss often worry that frequent shampooing aggravates the loss. This is not true. Indeed, the reverse may be correct in male pattern baldness. Dr Ronald Rizer and colleagues at the New York University Medical Center have found that the scalp sebum contains androgens and claimed that these may re-enter the scalp and aggravate male pattern baldness if the scalp is not regularly shampooed.

6

PATCHY BALDNESS

This condition affects about 0.1% of the general population and appears suddenly as one to three bald patches. There are usually no symptoms and the person may be unaware of the hair loss until this is pointed out to them.

The patches may be white, smooth and completely bald or there may be black dots (representing broken-off hair stumps) or "exclamation mark" hairs (these are hair stumps with a thin base and a thicker brushlike end). Exclamation mark hairs are a sign that hair loss is still active and that the patch may extend in size.

There have been a few cases of alopecia areata affecting pigmented hairs alone and causing them to fall out, leaving only the white hairs. This can cause hair to "turn white overnight." Historical examples are Sir Thomas More and Marie Antoinette, whose hairs were reported to have suddenly turned white before their executions.

Alopecia areata usually affects the scalp in patches (Figs. 12 and 13). However, in a few patients, these may enlarge

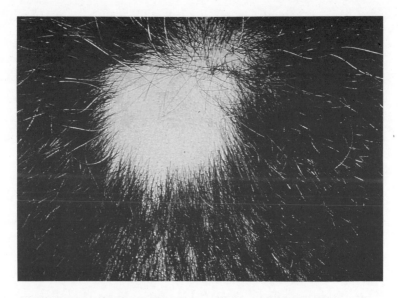

Fig. 12   A single typical patch of alopecia

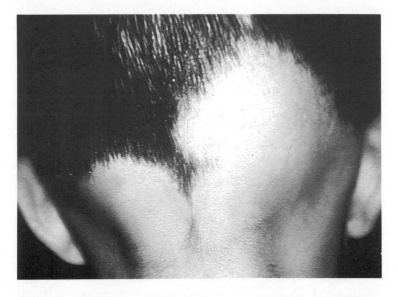

Fig. 13   Alopecia in child shows beginning of ophiasis

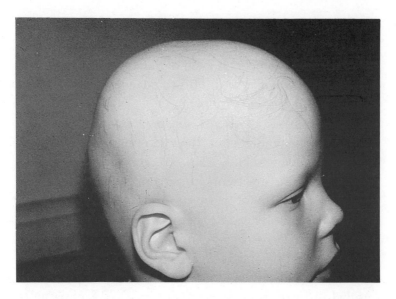

Fig. 14   Alopecia universalis: note absence of eyebrow
and eyelash

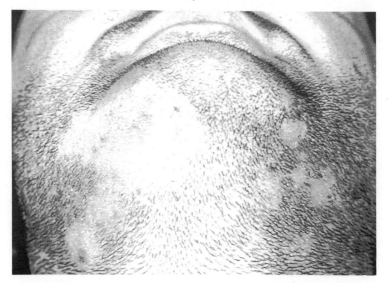

Fig. 15   Multiple patches of alopecia in beard region

rapidly and merge together to produce complete baldness of the scalp—a condition known as *alopecia totalis*. Sometimes the alopecia is even more severe and spreads to affect the body hair as well. This causes a universal alopecia or *alopecia universalis* (Fig. 14).

In about 10% of patients, alopecia areata affects areas other than the scalp such as the eyelashes, eyebrows, beard (Fig. 15), pubic and body hair. Alopecia areata may affect the nails in 10% of patients, causing pitting and ridging. A similar proportion of patients also suffer from atopic conditions such as *atopic dermatitis* (eczema), *asthma* (wheezy breathing) or *allergic rhinitis* (itchy, runny or stuffy nose).

Most cases of alopecia areata occur between the ages of 20-40 years but any age, race or sex may be affected. A family history of this case is present in 10-20% of patients, suggesting that the tendency to develop alopecia areata may be inherited. Identical twins have been reported to develop it on identical areas of their head at around the same time.

The cause of alopecia areata is unknown. The currently favoured theory is the autoimmune theory (meaning self allergy). According to this theory, the body's lymphocytes (a type of white cells) attack the hair follicles and cause hair to fall. Support for this theory comes from the following observations:

1) Microscopic examination of the affected skin (scalp biopsy) shows hair follicles surrounded by large numbers of lymphocytes. Lymphocytes are normally involved in immune reactions and their aggregation around the hair follicles suggest that they are participating in an immune reaction against the hair follicles.

2) Alopecia areata is frequently associated with other diseases suspected of having an autoimmune basis such as vitiligo (milky white patches of depigmented skin), thyroid disease, Addison's disease, pernicious anaemia and diabetes.
3) Steroids and other drugs which suppress the immune system appear to help alopecia areata.

However, why alopecia areata normally affects only certain patches and not the whole scalp defies explanation.

Emotional stress is believed to play a role. Patients with alopecia areata sometimes recall a sudden stressful event a few weeks before its onset. You may recall that the hair of Sir Thomas More and Marie Antoinette suddenly turned white on news of their impending executions. It is believed that alopecia areata affected the pigmented hairs, causing them to fall off, leaving only the white hairs.

Although stress may play a role in precipitating alopecia areata, it is not the cause. That stress may precipitate alopecia areata is still not inconsistent with the autoimmune theory because stress is known to cause alterations in immune function.

In the past, doctors went to the extent of saying that alopecia areata was entirely due to "nerves." This is not only unkind but also scientifically incorrect.

One reason could be that some patients with alopecia areata appeared neurotic or depressed about their alopecia. However, this is understandable because hair loss is very distressing, even to the most stable of characters.

Another reason could be that doctors those days were unable to offer much treatment and used that as an excuse for not treating them. This is certainly not the case today.

Modern doctors understand alopecia areata better and have more effective treatments at their disposal.

Diagnosis

Alopecia areata has to be differentiated from other conditions that cause patchy hair loss such as trichotillomania, tinea capitis (scalp ringworm) and secondary syphilis.

In alopecia areata, the scalp skin appears normal and exclamation mark hairs or black dots representing hairs broken off close to the scalp may be seen. If required, the diagnosis of alopecia areata can be confirmed with a scalp biopsy (see page 82).

Treatment

Less severe cases of alopecia areata usually recover on their own, but this may take as long as six months and sometimes as long as five years. Unfortunately, it is not possible to accurately predict which patients are going to improve on their own and which are not. Treatment can hasten recovery and is therefore desirable for psychological as well as cosmetic reasons. Below are some of the treatments available:

Intralesional steroids

This involves injecting steroids directly into the bald patches at monthly intervals until regrowth becomes evident, which may take six to 12 weeks. The regrown hairs may be light or white in colour but will darken as they grow longer.

The injection is no more painful than injections elsewhere and there is no danger of the injection injuring the brain, which is well protected by the skull. Intralesional steroids may not be suitable for children because of the pain.

Topical (applied) steroids

Strong steroids applied to the bald areas twice daily have been reported to produce regrowth in some patients. However, response is slow, taking sometimes up to six months and it is difficult to know whether response is due to treatment or the natural tendency of the condition to improve. Still, topical steroids are convenient, painless and worth a trial, especially in young children who may be fearful of injections.

Oral steroids

Steroids given by mouth are extremely effective, but the problem is that hair often falls out when treatment is discontinued. Therefore, treatment has to be continued until spontaneous remission takes place, which may take six months or more.

Prolonged treatment may cause side effects such as weight gain, easy skin bruising, upset stomach, bone thinning and muscle weakness. Therefore, oral steroids are usually only prescribed for severe cases of alopecia areata, alopecia totalis, alopecia universalis and for unresponsive patients who are psychologically very disturbed by their hair loss. Close supervision by the doctor is necessary because of side effects.

Minoxidil

Minoxidil lotion was originally developed for the treatment of male pattern baldness. A few small-scale studies suggest that minoxidil can induce regrowth in 50-80% of patients with alopecia areata. However, these results may not be that impressive when it is remembered that a significant proportion of patients regrow hair spontaneously anyway. Moreover, minoxidil does not work very well in patients with severe alopecia areata, alopecia totalis and alopecia universalis, which are genuinely difficult to treat.

Nonetheless, minoxidil is a new alternative available and may be tried in patients who are not keen on intralesional injections or in those who have not responded to other treatments. Minoxidil is believed to work by directly stimulating the hair follicles or modifying the immune reaction responsible for the hair loss.

Topical irritants
These are applied to the bald areas to irritate and stimulate hibernating hair follicles to produce hair again. Dithranol cream used for treating a skin condition known as psoriasis (see chapter 7) has been used with some success and regrowth has been reported in a few patients after about two months.

The disadvantage of dithranol is that the cream is somewhat irritating to the skin and causes itching and, occasionally, burning. It may also stain the clothes and skin. A variety of other irritants such as phenol, benzyl benzoate, sodium lauryl sulphate and croton oil have also been used. Irritants have to be applied regularly to maintain the irritation. Treatment is uncomfortable and hence not very popular with patients.

Ultraviolet-B light
Ultraviolet-B from an artificial light source has also been used to induce a mild sunburn on the bald areas. It is

believed that the mild sunburn irritates and stimulates the hair follicles into producing hair again. However, this treatment is inconvenient because the patient has to go to the clinic regularly for treatment.

Topical allergens

Instead of irritation, this method uses allergens (substances that cause an allergic reaction) to stimulate the follicles into producing hair. A number of allergens have been used, for example, DNCB (dinitrochlorbenzene), SADBE (squaric acid dibutylester), diphencyprone, poison ivy resin and primula leaves. Application of any one of these will induce allergy in most people.

If the same substance (allergen) is applied to the skin again, an allergic reaction will develop at the site of application. Repeated applications maintain the reaction, and about 25-50% of patients with severe alopecia areata have shown regrowth three to six months later.

It is believed that the allergic reaction induces the production of a group of lymphocytes known as suppressor-T cells which suppress the immune reaction responsible for the hair loss.

Topical allergens definitely work because some patients who have been totally bald for years have regrown hair. The problem is the reaction can be very uncomfortable and at times associated with painful swelling of the lymph glands in the neck and fever. DNCB is less popular now because laboratory tests show that it may be cancer-causing.

PUVA

Psoralen plus ultraviolet light-A, normally used for treating psoriasis, has also been used in patients with alopecia areata.

This treatment is repeated two to five times a week at the clinic for a total of about 20 treatments. The results have been variable with some doctors reporting benefit and others reporting none.

Like ultraviolet-B light, this treatment requires the patient to go to the clinic regularly for treatment. Special precautions have to be taken to avoid direct sunlight for several hours after treatment. PUVA has a depleting effect on Langerhan cells (another type of cell that is involved in immune reactions) and this somehow encourages hair growth.

Isoprinosine

This is an immunomodulatory drug (a drug which has effects on the immune system). It has been reported to induce regrowth in patients with alopecia areata who have laboratory evidence of altered immunity. Isoprinosine may cause an increase in uric acid, causing gout; so monitoring of uric acid levels is a necessary precaution during treatment.

Cyclosporin

Cyclosporin is a drug used to prevent the rejection of transplanted organs. It suppresses the immune system and also causes hair growth as a side effect.

Oral cyclosporin has been reported to induce regrowth in some patients with alopecia areata. It may work by suppressing the immune reaction that is causing the hair loss or by directly stimulating hair follicle growth.

Because cyclosporin is toxic when taken by mouth, doctors have tried using topical cyclosporin instead. Unfortunately, only mild regrowth was observed. Like in male pattern baldness, this may be related to the inability of cyclosporin to penetrate the skin and reach the follicles.

Doctors are experimenting with other formulations in an attempt to improve the penetration of cyclosporin into the skin.

Outcome

The outcome of alopecia areata is, unfortunately, very unpredictable. As a general guide, 50% of patients will recover their hair within six to 12 months. Unfavourable signs include alopecia areata of greater than one year's duration, extensive alopecia areata, alopecia totalis and alopecia universalis, and a history of atopy (asthma, allergic rhinitis or atopic dermatitis).

Ophiasis, a form of alopecia areata affecting the back of the head and spreading in a band along the scalp margins, also has a poor outlook (Fig. 13). After full recovery, there is a 40-50% chance of a relapse within five years.

7

TEMPORARY HAIR LOSS AND OTHER DISORDERS

Temporary hair loss (telogen effluvium)

You may remember from chapter 3 that anagen hairs grow for a period of five years before entering telogen. Telogen is the resting stage which lasts 2-5 months, after which the hairs are shed.

Normally, about 85% of the hairs are in anagen and 15% are in telogen. Under certain circumstances, however, many anagen hairs are prematurely pushed into telogen and at the end of five months (sometimes less), these hairs are all shed. Such a condition is known as telogen effluvium (*effluvium* in Latin means to flow out). In this condition, between 30 and 50% of the hairs are in telogen and these can be lost over a matter of a few days. Hair loss occurs in handfuls and can be very alarming. There are several causes of telogen effluvium:

- Prolonged high fever (ie., typhoid, malaria)
- Post-delivery

- Surgery
- Haemorrhage
- Crash diet
- Emotional crises (i.e., bereavement)
- Drugs, including birth control pills

Patients with telogen effluvium usually complain of sudden and excessive hair loss to begin with. Thinning becomes obvious when 40-50% of hair in one area are lost. This is different from patients with male pattern baldness who complain of gradual thinning, and those with alopecia areata who complain of the sudden onset of a few bald patches.

Telogen effluvium is a temporary form of hair loss. After the stimulus has passed off or is removed, hair will regrow. Full recovery may take six months.

Karen, 32, started losing large quantities of hair about two months after delivering her second child. Examination confirmed that she suffered from telogen effluvium related to childbirth. I reassured Karen that the hair loss was temporary and recommended that she wear a wig until her hair regrew.

I saw Karen again three months and then six months later. On the latter occasion, all her hair had regrown and she was able to do without her wig.

Hair breakage

Hair breakage is different from true hair loss, in which the hair is lost together with its root.

Hair breakage may be caused by:

Improper hair care. Excessive bleaching, permanent

71

waving, hot combing, hair ironing and straightening can weaken hair and cause it to break easily.

Hairstyles. Ponytails, tight braids, corn rows, buns and curling the hair excessively tight may pull them out by the roots and cause *traction alopecia.* If the hairstyle is continued, permanent hair loss may occur.

Ringworm of the scalp (tinea capitis) produces bald patches with broken-off hair stumps. The underlying skin is usually red and scaly and the hairs can be easily pulled out (Fig. 7).

Structural defects of the hair. Many of these are inherited and appear during early childhood. *Monolethrix* (beaded hair) and *pili torti* (twisted hair) are just two examples. In these conditions, hairs break off a few centimetres from the scalp surface.

Trichotillomania (compulsive hair pulling, see Fig. 6). This causes patches of broken hairs with stubbled ends. It usually affects children and women and is due to underlying emotional stress. In adults, trichotillomania is often caused by severe psychological problems; help from a psychiatrist may be necessary. In children, helping them gain some insight into the cause of hair loss and reassurance is all that is necessary. Permanent hair loss may develop if the hair-pulling habit is continued.

Split ends (trichoptilosis)

This is a common problem in people who keep very long hair. Split ends are harmless. Conditioners help, but the best way to deal with them is to cut the split ends off.

Dandruff (seborrhoeic dermatitis)

This is a common condition affecting areas of the skin rich in sebaceous (oil) glands, namely the face and scalp and, to a lesser extent, the upper chest and back.

Ordinarily, seborrhoeic dermatitis just causes flaking of the scalp, or dandruff. Sometimes, it is more extensive and spreads to the eyebrows, the folds on the sides of the nose, behind the ears, the upper chest and the back.

There may be associated itching. Its exact cause is unknown, but there is increasing evidence now that it is in some way related to an overgrowth of a normal skin fungus, pityrosporon yeast.

Dandruff can be controlled with medicated shampoos, like those with zinc pyrithione, salicylic acid, tar or selenium sulphide. These are over-the-counter (OTC) products which can be bought off the pharmacy shelf.

More stubborn cases require the application of steroid creams, gels or lotions which have to be prescribed by the doctor. Anti-fungal shampoos such as ketoconazole and econazole shampoos have recently been introduced into the market. They are more effective than conventional medicated shampoos but rather expensive. Their effectiveness support a fungal cause of dandruff.

Dandruff is not contagious. You cannot catch dandruff from others and neither will you spread it to them. Dandruff is quite common and can be found coincidentally in people with hair loss. It does not cause hair loss. However, it can cause scalp itchiness and vigorous scratching may aggravate the hair loss. Treatment is, therefore, important.

Psoriasis

This is a chronic skin disorder which causes well-defined

red patches covered by thick, adherent, silvery scales. It may affect any part of the skin, particularly the scalp, elbows and knees.

On the scalp, the scales may get very thick and stick to the hair. However, alopecia is unusual unless complicated by bacterial infection.

In psoriasis, the skin cells divide about seven times faster than normal. They do not have time to mature properly and are more sticky than normal. As a result, they stick to one another, forming heaps of scales characteristic of psoriasis. Its cause is unknown, but heredity plays an important role. It is not contagious.

There is no cure for psoriasis, but it can be controlled. Scalp psoriasis can be treated with tar or salicylic acid-containing shampoos, steroid or tar lotions and gels, and dithranol preparations (these are derived from tar).

PUVA is useful for treating psoriasis involving a large part of the body. The patient takes a light-sensitizing medicine—psoralen—and is exposed for a few minutes to ultraviolet-A light about two hours later. This treatment is repeated two to five times a week at the clinic.

Twenty to 25 treatments are necessary before there is clearance or marked improvement. PUVA has also been used to treat alopecia areata (see page 68).

8
DIAGNOSING HAIR LOSS

Localized hair loss which causes bald patches is easily recognized as abnormal; you should see a doctor immediately. This is because some conditions that cause patchy hair loss such as discoid lupus erythematosus, lichen planus and scleroderma may go on to produce scarring. Once scarring sets in, there is no prospect of any hair growing again.

Clumps of hair falling out as in telogen effluvium is so alarming that the patient usually wastes no time in consulting the doctor. The problem lies in detecting gradual hair loss of the type seen in male pattern baldness, particularly in its early stages. Thinning will eventually become obvious when 40-50% of the hairs in one area are lost, but the recognition of early hair loss is important because early treatment is more likely to be effective.

Not every patient that consults the doctor for hair loss is suffering from true hair loss. For example, people who brush their hair for the first time may notice an alarming number of hairs in the hair brush. This is quite normal.

I've also seen women with long hair who come to the clinic in a state of great anxiety, concerned that they are going bald. When asked how they arrived at such a conclusion, they would gather their hair behind the head and say, "Look how thin it is; it used to be very much thicker."

The truth, of course, is long hairs tend to break easily and what is gathered together behind the head are only the long ones. These women do not suffer from true hair loss. A change of hairstyle is all that is necessary. More objective tests for hair loss are necessary. Below are two examples:

Shed Hair Count

This involves collecting hairs lost in combs, hair brushes, showers, basins, on clothes and pillow cases over three days (remember to clear these areas of hair beforehand). Each day's collection is carefully placed in an envelope and labelled accordingly.

After completing three days' collection, examine the hairs with a magnifying glass and separate those with from those without roots. Those without roots are indicative of hair breakage whereas those with roots indicate true hair loss. Divide each by three to obtain the daily rate of hair breakage or hair loss.

Normal hair loss may range from 50 to 100 per day, but for purposes of this test, 50 is considered to be the cut-off point. Any loss beyond that may indicate excessive hair loss. But relax! It does not mean that you are on the verge of baldness. Consult a doctor for proper diagnosis.

Hair breakage is not a serious problem because the hair follicles are not damaged and hair has the potential to grow again. However, hair breakage indicates improper hair care and this calls for some modification in your hair care routine. If you lose more than 30 broken hairs a day, see your doctor or hairdresser for advice.

Unfortunately, collecting hairs lost in the shower and basin can be a rather messy business and some patience is required to count the number of hairs lost.

Long hairs are also difficult to count because they often get entangled. A much simpler screening test for excessive hair loss is the pull test described below.

The Pull Test
Ensure that you have not washed or brushed your hair during the preceding 24 hours. In this test, about 10 hairs are grasped at the base with the thumb, index and middle fingers and firm pulling pressure is exerted while the hairs slip through the fingers.

You will remember from chapter 3 that 85% of hair are in anagen and 15% in telogen. For practical purposes, however, doctors regard 20% as the maximum proportion of hairs that should be in telogen. If 20% of the hairs are in telogen, then not more than two hairs should be pulled out from a clump of 10.

The test result would indicate, therefore, that hair loss is abnormal when *more than two hairs with roots* are pulled out. It can be repeated over different areas of the scalp to detect where the abnormal hair loss is occuring.

Like the shed hair count, an abnormal pull test only indicates possible hair loss. More objective testing by the doctor is required to confirm whether or not you are losing excessive hair.

Diagnosing the type of hair loss is not as straightforward as you may think. The doctor relies heavily on your history and his physical and laboratory findings. Let us examine each of these to give you an idea of what to expect when you consult a dermatologist (skin specialist).

History

Your hair history is extremely useful for diagnosing hair problems, so it is important that you provide all the necessary information. Below is a list of questions, adapted from *Diseases of the Hair and Nail* by H. P. Baden, that the doctor may ask.

Present hair problem
- What is the nature of the problem?
- Which areas of the scalp are affected?
- Are other body areas affected?
- When did the problem begin?
- How many hairs do you lose each day?
- Is it coming off at the roots or breaking off?
- Is it stable, improving or worsening?
- Have you noticed changes in your skin, nails or teeth?
- Do you pull or twirl your hair?

Health problems
- List past illnesses, operations and hospitalizations.
- Do you have any present health problems?
- Has there been any significant weight change, emotional crisis or life changes (i.e., marriage, divorce, shifting house, job changes) during the six months preceding the hair loss?
- Date of last pregnancy.

- Have you ever suffered from hair loss following delivery?
- Have you been on birth control pills before? If so, give dates.
- Have you noticed any change in menstruation?
- Do you suffer from diabetes or thyroid problems?
- Has there been any change in your tolerance to heat and cold?
- Do you have any unusual dietary habits?

Present hair care

1) Cleansing:
- Shampoo—what brand and frequency of use.
- Conditioner—what brand and frequency of use.

2) Hair setting—do you use any of the following, and if so, how frequent?
- Permanent wave
- Electric hair-rollers
- Curling irons
- Hot combs
- Hair straighteners

3) Hair colouring:
- Type—temporary tints/semi-permanent dyes/ permanent dyes
- Frequency
- Do you bleach your hair?

4) Hair styling:
- Describe your usual hairstyle.
- Do you wear buns, braids (corn rowing), ponytails?

- Do you use elastics?
- Do you brush your hair every day?
- Do you use a hair dryer? If so, indicate whether you blow till the hair is half dried or completely dry?
- Do you use hair sprays? If so, give names.

Family history

Are there any illnesses that seem to run in your family? Do any of the following suffer from hair problems? List down the ages of your parents, brothers and sisters and describe the condition of their hair.

Examination

This is the next step. The doctor conducts a careful physical examination, paying special attention to your hair and scalp.

The pattern of baldness is very important. Patchy hair loss may indicate alopecia areata, secondary syphilis, tinea capitis or trichotillomania. In men, thinning of the crown and a receding hairline is indicative of male pattern baldness; but in women, there may be thinning of the crown alone.

Diffuse hair loss may be the result of telogen effluvium, iron deficiency and thyroid disorders. The state of the scalp and hair is also noted. Exclamation mark hairs occuring in a bald patch are diagnostic of alopecia areata.

Broken-off hair stumps of different lengths may indicate trichotillomania or secondary syphilis. Tinea capitis may also cause broken-off hair stumps, but in this condition the scalp also shows redness, scaliness and in severe cases even swelling, inflammation and pus formation.

The doctor may also illuminate the area with a Wood's lamp. In some forms of tinea capitis, a green or pale yellow fluorescence may be seen. Hairs broken off a few millimetres from a normal-looking scalp may indicate a structural defect of the hair such as monolethrix and pili torti.

Laboratory tests

Additional tests may sometimes be necessary to confirm the diagnosis. These may include:

Blood tests. This may be done to detect iron deficiency, thyroid disease, excessive androgen production, syphilis and discoid lupus erythematosus.

Microscopy. This allows the doctor to identify structural defects and fungal infections.

Culture. This is used to detect fungal infections. However, the result takes six weeks to return, limiting its usefulness.

Anagen-telogen ratio. In this test, between 20 and 30 hairs are carefully plucked to include their roots and examined under a microscope.

Anagen and telogen hairs can be identified and their number and the ratio of anagen to telogen hairs (A:T ratio) determined. As explained earlier, doctors regard 20% as the maximum proportion of hairs in telogen. Using this figure, the normal A:T ratio should be at least 80:20 (80% anagen:20% telogen) or 4:1. It is reduced in telogen effluvium and in areas affected by male pattern baldness.

Hair density. This is done by shaving a small area of the scalp about four centimetres above the ear. The area is then stamped with a biopsy punch, an instrument of eight millimetre in diameter, giving a circle of 0.5 square centimetre in area. The number of hairs (not the follicle openings) within the circle is counted with the aid of a magnifying glass, and the number of hairs per square centimetre calculated. The normal number is 150 per square centimetre.

Length of hair growth. An area of the scalp is shaved and the length of hair measured a month later. The norm is 1-1.2 centimetre per month. The same area of the scalp used for measuring hair density can also be used. This test is also useful for reassuring the patient that hair is growing.

Scalp biopsy. This involves removing a piece of scalp tissue and examining it under a microscope. The area to be biopsied is first anaesthetized to numb the pain. It is useful for the diagnosis of many scalp and hair disorders. The discomfort is minimal and there is no risk of injuring underlying structures such as the skull bones or the brain.

Apart from examining and conducting tests, the doctor is also there to answer any queries that you may have; so make the best use of your time with him or her. Hair loss is a distressing condition and may cause a variety of psychological problems. The doctor can counsel and provide psychological support if this is required.

9
PUTTING HAIR BACK (WIGS AND SURGERY)

Wigs

People often frown at the thought of having to wear wigs and regard them as unattractive and unnatural. This may be said of wigs in the past but most modern-day wigs are very well made and attractive.

It may interest you to know that wigs were very fashionable during the days of the pharoahs. Women then used to shave their heads and had several wigs, each to suit her attire for the social occasion. There is no need to be superstitious about wearing wigs. They will not cause hair loss or stop hair from growing.

There are two types of wigs—one which covers a portion of the scalp (commonly called a hairpiece) and the other which covers the entire scalp.

Wigs may be made of synthetic material (acrylic) or human hair. Each has its advantages and disadvantages. Wigs made of human hair look more natural but they are rather expensive because human hair is difficult to obtain.

Few people are willing to grow hair long enough to be sold to wig manufacturers. Hair also have to be washed and styled regularly and are not as lasting as synthetic ones.

Synthetic wigs may not be "natural," but they can be extremely attractive. Some of the more expensive ones can even be styled or dyed to match the remaining hair on the scalp.

When purchasing wigs, it is very important to check the material used for the base. Solid plastic bases are not suitable for hot humid climates because they make the scalp very hot, greasy and uncomfortable. Fibre mesh bases allow ventilation and are more comfortable, but they tend to get stretched out of shape with wear.

Attaching wigs to the scalp

One problem with wigs is that they sometimes fall off, much to the embarrassment of the wearer. A number of methods for securing wigs are available:

Hair weaving

This consists of weaving the remaining hair to form an anchor to which the wig can be tied. The problem with this method is that there must be some hair left to weave.

It is suitable for male pattern baldness in men since there is at least a horseshoe rim of hair left, but it is not suitable for people who are completely bald.

Another problem with hair weaving is that the attachment loosens as the natural hair grows longer, requiring repeated weavings every six months or so. Still, hair weaving is done extremely well by some professional hair clinics and is worth considering.

Suture implant

This involves inserting steel sutures (stitches) into strategic areas on the scalp and the wig is then tied to these. The procedure is done under local anaesthesia. The problem with suture implants is that infection may occur at the entry points of the sutures. Another disadvantage is that you cannot remove the wig in public for swimming and sports as the sutures will show.

Tunnel graft

In this method, skin grafts are used to create tunnels of skin on the front and back of the scalp. Velcro straps or clips are then used to attach the wig to the tunnel grafts. There is no risk of infection. The procedure is done under local anaesthesia.

Tapes and adhesives

Special hypoallergenic (less allergy causing) tapes and adhesives can be used to attach wigs directly onto the scalp. They are convenient, easy to use and completely pain free.

Carol, 34, suffered from alopecia totalis for three years. She wore a scarf to hide the baldness but had resisted wearing a wig all this while. She had spent a lot of time and money on treatment and almost everything had been tried to no avail.

I thought the best strategy was to get her to wear a wig, explaining that it could be viewed as a temporary measure to conceal hair loss until such time that her hair grew back again. I explained that wigs nowadays were very well made and attractive and certainly a lot more "natural" than wearing a scarf. She agreed to give it a try.

I started Carol on dithranol cream 0.5% which she continued for four months without improvement. In the meantime, she had started to wear an acrylic wig. She found the wig very attractive and even started attending social functions, something she had stopped doing since she became bald.

When I saw Carol again, she informed me that she didn't want to try any other messy treatments (referring to the dithranol) and was quite happy wearing her wig. One year later, she returned to find out whether there was anything new in the treatment of hair loss.

She mentioned that her hair grew for a while and she was able to do without the wig during that time. Unfortunately, her hair started to fall out again. However, she had no hesitation about wearing her wig the second time around.

Surgery

Unlike wigs, surgery is only suitable for some types of baldness such as male pattern baldness and for hair loss due to scarring (for example, after burns).

Surgery is feasible because the hair follicles retain their characteristics regardless of where they are transplanted to. This is why grafts taken from the back of the scalp and transplanted to a bald area affected by male pattern baldness do not also succumb to male pattern baldness.

Surgery is performed by plastic surgeons and some dermatologists. However, it is an expensive and protracted procedure and not every patient is suitable for surgery. The surgeon will assess each patient individually and decide whether surgery is the answer.

Surgery will improve the appearance, but whether the improvement is acceptable to the patient is another matter. Your expectations of improvement must coincide with the improvement that surgery can bring about.

If your expectations are too high, then you are likely to be disappointed with the results of surgery. You cannot also expect surgery to change other aspects of your life, such as career advancement, wealth and friends; these depend on other factors, not appearance alone.

Below are some of the surgical treatments available:

Punch grafting
This involves taking cylindrical grafts of the hair-bearing skin (usually from the back of the scalp) and transplanting them onto the bald areas where similar or slightly smaller-sized holes have been punched out (Fig. 16).

Several sessions are required and at each session 80 to 100 grafts may be done. The procedure can be performed under local anaesthesia. Grafts are obtained with a biopsy punch (which works like a cookie cutter). The hair on the graft will fall off but new hair will begin to grow after three to four months. Punch grafting is probably the best form of surgery for male pattern baldness.

Strip grafting
This is similar to the above except a strip of hair-bearing scalp is removed and transplanted to the bald area. The wound left behind is then closed with sutures.

Scalp reduction
This involves removing a strip of bald scalp and then stitching the edges together. Scalp reduction (Fig. 17)

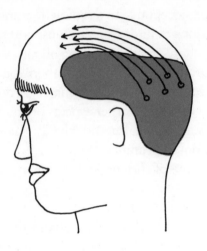

Fig. 16 Punch grafting

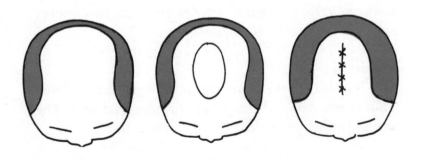

Fig. 17 Scalp reduction

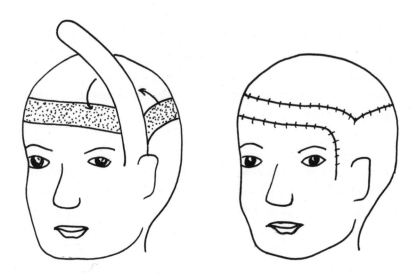

Fig. 18 Transposition flap

reduces the size of the bald patch. The width of the strip that can be removed depends on the laxity of the scalp; a lax scalp will allow a larger strip to be removed.

Scalp reduction is commonly performed prior to transplantation to reduce the amount of graft required. It is particularly useful for people who do not have much hair left for grafting. Scalp reduction can be done under local anaesthesia. Another benefit of scalp reduction is that it gives the face a mild face lift.

Transposition flaps

Transposition flaps were originally used for the treatment of baldness resulting from burns and other scarring diseases. The same procedure has also been used for treating male pattern baldness. It involves raising a pedicle flap of hair-bearing skin (a flap of scalp with a stalk or pedicle still attached to it) and removing a strip of skin from the bald area. The flap is then rotated around its stalk and stitched into place on the bald area (Fig. 18).

Transposition flaps are useful because they can reposition large areas of hair bearing scalp onto the bald areas. However, the procedure needs great technical skill in order to produce good results. A more complicated type of transposition flap is the Juri Flap, named after its inventor. This allows even larger areas of hair-bearing skin to be transposed, but even greater skill is required.

Hair implants

This consists of inserting natural or synthetic hairs into the scalp. The ends of the hairs are barbed or knotted. Unfortunately, they still fall out and infection and inflammation commonly occurs. Avoid this treatment!

10
HAIR CARE

Proper hair care is important for normal hair, particularly for hair that is thinning. Unfortunately, not many people understand the basics of hair care and get lured by advertisements into using products that may not be suitable. Let us examine some aspects of hair care so that you can use hair products and styles to the best advantage.

Shampooing
Shampoos are cleansing agents rather like ordinary soaps. Indeed, shampoos in the past were soap based, but these had the disadvantage of being affected by hard water. They caused a scum deposit and made hair look dull. Modern shampoos contain synthetic detergents and work equally well in hard or soft water.

There are essentially three types of shampoos available in the market. They are (1) shampoos for dry hair, (2) shampoos for normal hair and (3) shampoos for oily hair. There are other subclassifications, but these are unnecessary and confusing. The difference essentially lies in the amount of oil (lanolin, natural or mineral oil) added to them.

Shampoos for dry hair contain oil whereas those for normal or oily hair generally do not. It is helpful to choose the right shampoo for your type of hair.

If your hair looks greasy and matted together, then use a shampoo for oily hair. If these prove too drying even for oily hair, use a normal hair formula and wash more frequently or double wash. It should be remembered that the basic purpose of all shampoos is to clean the hair and all shampoos do this very well. Since they are all equally effective, you might like to choose the best-smelling one, remembering that price is not necessarily an indication of quality.

Some shampoos are labelled "acid-balanced" or "pH-balanced." The detergents found in all shampoos are alkaline (they have to be, otherwise they will not clean) and open the imbrications (spaces) in the cuticle so that hair gets entangled easily. This effect is minimized by acid- or pH-balanced shampoos.

Another group of shampoos available in the market are called medicated shampoos. These contain substances that help itchy scalp conditions such as dandruff or seborrhoeic dermatitis and psoriasis.

Despite the name, medicated shampoos do not contain medicine for the hair and will not help hair to grow; neither will they cause hair loss. They can be safely used to treat people with hair loss who have co-existing scalp conditions such as seborrhoeic dermatitis or psoriasis. Medicated shampoos are generally more drying and a conditioner may be used if this is a problem.

All sorts of claims have been made by the manufacturers of shampoos and hundreds of healthful-sounding substances are added to entice the consumer into choosing their products. In truth, shampoos only clean hair; they do not nourish hair. All the nourishment for the hair is provided by the blood vessels around the hair follicles and nothing applied to the scalp will affect the follicles below.

Shampooing is not harmful even for people with hair loss. Regular shampooing keeps the scalp and hair clean, healthy-looking and comfortable. It may also help male pattern baldness by removing locally-produced androgens from the scalp (see page 58). These androgens are believed to contibute towards male pattern baldness.

Recently, a number of 2-in-1 shampoos have been introduced into the market. These contain the additional conditioner. Frankly, I believe it is better to use conditioners separately after shampooing because the detergent in 2-in-1 shampoos probably wash away most of the conditioner.

How you use the shampoo is also important for getting the best out of the shampoo. Wet the hair first, then pour a 20-cent-size dollop of shampoo into your hand. Spread it between the fingers and then work the shampoo into the scalp. It is incorrect to pour shampoo directly on to the scalp because cleaning will be uneven with some parts getting more shampoo than others.

Rinse off thoroughly afterwards. Remember that the cleansing ability is not related to the amount of lather the shampoo produces. Some shampoos clean exceptionally well even though they produce very little lather.

Conditioning

Shampoos are just cleansing agents and really all they are meant to be. That is why conditioners were developed; they help hair that is dry and unmanageable, seal split ends and give hair a little body.

There are basically three types: (1) conditioners to reduce static and prevent the fly-away look, (2) conditioners that give body and temporarily glue split ends together and (3) conditioners that replace the oils removed by the detergents in shampoos.

The first type contains quarternary ammonium compounds to reduce static. The second contains hydrolyzed animal proteins which coat the hair with protein and give it extra thickness. They also help to fill up any cracks in the cuticle caused by perming and bleaching. The third contains oils which coat hair, making it look shiny and lustrous and preventing it from getting entangled and breaking off during combing.

Another product that works like a conditioner is the acid rinse. You may recall that shampoos are alkaline and ruffle up the cuticles, causing hair to get entangled. The acid rinse neutralizes the alkalinity of shampoos, reducing static and thereby reducing the fly-away look. It also makes the hair smoother and more manageable. Lemon juice and vinegar may be used to make a simple acid rinse.

Most conditioners nowadays contain many of the substances mentioned earlier so that one conditioner can prevent the fly-away look, give hair fullness and make them manageable as well as temporarily seal split ends.

Thickeners

These contain vinyls and waxes which coat the hair and make them look thick. Thickeners are applied to damp hair and combed or brushed into it. The hair is then allowed to dry completely. A final brush fluffs up the hair again.

Hair sprays

These help to keep hair in place. There are basically two types of hair sprays. The alcohol-based hair spray, also called soft hold spray formula, hardens the hair as the alcohol evaporates. The most common ingredient in these is something called SD alcohol 40. SD means specially denatured or undrinkable. The plastic or vinyl-based hair spray, also called hard hold hair spray formula, coats the hair with a layer and keeps it in position when it hardens.

At the moment, there is great concern about the destruction of the Earth's ozone layer by chlorofluorocarbons (CFCs). If you are concerned, use CFC-free hair sprays.

Hair drying

Avoid vigorous towelling, but gently pat the hair dry with a towel and then comb the hair with a *wide* tooth comb. Never use a brush on wet hair. You can then allow the hair to dry naturally (which is preferred) or use a hair dryer.

When using a hair dryer, set it to a slower and cooler setting and hold it at least six inches away. Move the hair dryer from spot to spot and continue blowing until the hair is partially dry, then leave it to dry completely on its own. Do not blow hair until it is completely dry as this tends to overdry and cause it to become brittle or split at the ends.

Hairstyles

Hairstyles that exert traction on the hair—ponytails, corn rows, buns, etc.—are not a good idea for people with hair loss problems. Other styles can be used to conceal hair loss.

One of the most popular methods used by men to conceal hair loss is what I call the "up and over." In this method, hair is grown long on one side and then combed over and upwards to cover the bald area. In my view, this method is unsatisfactory and probably attracts more attention to the hair loss. One would be better off seeking the help of a hairdresser.

The professional hairdresser can recommend an appropriate style to disguise areas of thinning or advise you on the use of conditioners and thickeners to help give hair a fuller look. There are other tricks which the hairdresser can do, such as highlighting certain areas to divert attention from areas of thinning.

The shape of our hair is determined by two types of linkages—hydrogen bonds which are weaker, and sulphur bonds which are stronger. These can be broken to make hair pliable so that it can be modelled to the desired shape.

Electric hair rollers and curling irons disrupt the hydrogen bonds. The first may be safe to use because the heat is not intense enough to hurt the hair. Curling irons on the other hand can definitely hurt your hair. The occasional use of curling irons just before a function does no real harm, but repeated use can damage the hair cuticle permanently. It is best to avoid them if you already suffer from hair loss.

The most popular form of hair waving used nowadays is permanent waving. It does not use heat and, hence, is also known as cold waving. It also gives a longer-lasting set to the hair.

In permanent waving, the sulphur bonds are first broken with solutions or foams containing thioglycollates (wave solution). The hair is then curled around rollers and left in place for a specified time. After that, the solution is neutralized by adding an oxidizing agent such as hydrogen peroxide. This causes the sulphur bonds to reform in their new position.

Great care must be taken when using permanent wave solutions; thioglycollates may damage hair and cause it to become brittle and break off. Damage to hair is a particular hazard when permanent waving is done at home. Permanent waving should be done not more than once every three months.

As a general rule, the hairstyle should be simple and easy to maintain. Avoid hairstyles such as ponytailing, corn rowing and tight braiding because these pull on hair, causing breakage and even permanent hair loss.

Keep the hair short because short hair is easier to manage and less likely to break. Short hair also looks thicker.

Hair sprays can be used safely to help hair hold its shape.

Hair colouring

Hair colourings have been used for centuries. The ancient Egyptians, Persians, Greeks and Romans used natural (vegetable) dyes such as henna. These were harmless on the hair. Nowadays, we use synthetic dyes which are extremely effective for colouring hair, but some may be damaging to the hair. There are three main types of synthetic hair dyes: (1) permanent dyes, (2) semi-permanent dyes and (3) temporary tints.

Permanent dyes are the most effective and lasting method' of colouring but are more difficult to apply and the most damaging of the types. They are also known as oxidation dyes because oxidation takes place within the hair.

The dye (paraphenylene diamine or PPD) is first of all mixed with a developer, hydrogen peroxide, and the mixture is applied. These chemicals enter the cortex, strip it of the pigment molecules and replace them with the new colour. The peroxide used in permanent dyes is rather damaging to the cuticle, and frequent dyeing can lead to hair breakage.

Another problem is that dyes such as PPD (which dyes hair black) can cause allergy. Most manufacturers recommend an allergy test beforehand. The freshly mixed dye is applied to cleansed skin behind the ear or on the upper inner arm and left for 24 hours. If redness, itching or swelling occurs, then the person is allergic to it.

However, allergies seem rare because millions of people are exposed to hair dyes and only a few develop them. This is fortunate because many salons do not carry out allergy tests beforehand.

Semi-permanent dyes are low molecular weight chemicals which can enter the hair and deposit there. They contain sulphur and thioglycollate instead of peroxide and are less damaging to the cuticle. Semi-permanent dyes last five or six shampooings.

Temporary tints are colour rinses which coat the hair with the desired colour. They do not contain peroxide or thioglycollate and will not hurt the hair. However, they can only lightly tint hair and are also washed off during shampooing. They are more useful for highlighting, brightening faded hair and toning down grey hair.

Dyeing dark hair a light colour requires the hair to be bleached first. This is done with a solution of hydrogen peroxide and an accelerator, persulphate. The accelerator increases the bleaching effect of hydrogen peroxide. After bleaching, a toner (light hair dye) is added. The bleaching process is even more damaging to the cuticle than permanent dyes.

The biggest controversy about hair dyes is whether or not they cause cancer. Artificial dyes used for colouring hair have been shown to cause cancer when fed in large amounts to rats. However, manufacturers of hair dyes argue that applying dyes on the scalp is not the same as eating them. Furthermore, there is no apparent link between women who use hair dyes and women who have cancer. Still, I think it is prudent for pregnant women and those with a family history of cancer to avoid using them.

Natural dyes are the safest hair dyes to use. These are derived from vegetables like henna, camomile, logwood, indigo and rhubarb. However, they do not offer versatility of colour like synthetic dyes and are generally less popular.

Temporary rinses are also harmless, but as explained earlier, these can only lightly tint hair and do not withstand shampooing. Moderation should be exercised when using other dyes, particularly if you suffer from hair loss. The dyeing process may damage the hair and cause breakage, further thinning hair.

SOME FINAL WORDS

You realize that this book does not offer you any miracle cure or a 100% effective treatment plan. The simple reason: there is no such thing; the sooner you learn this the better.

However, I do hope that this book has enabled you to understand more about your hair, how it grows, how it is lost and what can be done to help it grow. I hope it has reassured you that it is quite natural to feel distressed about losing hair but that it is equally important to learn how to cope with such stresses so that they do not get out of hand.

Before finishing, I would like to remind you of some rules that affect the health of your body, and your hair:

- Take a well-balanced diet.
- Reduce stress.
- Take adequate exercise.
- Ensure adequate rest and sleep.

I wish you every success in your fight against hair loss.

ABOUT THE AUTHOR

After graduating in 1978 in medicine from the Charing Cross Hospital Medical School in England, Dr Lim Kah-Beng went for further training in dermatology at the St John's Hospital for Diseases of the Skin in London. After completing his training, he returned to Singapore and spent six years working at the Middle Road Hospital before going into private practice.

Currently, he is a visiting consultant dermatologist to the National Skin Centre in Singapore. Dr Lim is also the author of *No More Pimples*, a self-care guide to acne treatment. He and his wife, Gaik, have two children, Siew Lin and Christopher.

BIBLIOGRAPHY

Baden, H.P.: "Diseases of the Hair and Nail," *Yearbook Medical Publishers*, Chicago, 1987; p. 116-117 and Table 11-1.

Bazzano, G.S., N. Terezakis and W. Galen: "Topical tretinoin for hair growth promotion," *Journal of the American Academy of Dermatology*, 1986; volume 15, p. 880.

Cotterill, J.A.: "Dermatological Non-Disease: A common and potentially fatal disturbance of cutaneous body image," *British Journal of Dermatology*, 1981; volume 104, p. 611.

Hamilton, J.B.: "Male hormone stimulation is prerequisite as an incitant in common baldness," *American Journal of Anatomy*, 1942; volume 71, p. 451.